skinny**smoothies**

skinny**smoothies**

101 Delicious Drinks
That Help You
Detox and Lose Weight

Shell Harris and Elizabeth Johnson

Da Capo
LIFE
LONG
A Member of the Perseus Books Group

Design by Cynthia Young

Cataloging-in-Publication data for this book is available from the Library of Congress.

First Da Capo Press edition 2012

ISBN: 978-0-7382-1600-3

Published by Da Capo Press

A Member of the Perseus Books Group

www.dacapopress.com

Da Capo Press books are available at special discounts for bulk purchases in the U.S. by corporations, institutions, and other organizations. For more information, please contact the Special Markets Department at the Perseus Books Group, 2300 Chestnut Street, Suite 200, Philadelphia, PA, 19103, or call (800) 810-4145, ext. 5000, or e-mail special.markets@perseusbooks.com.

10 9 8 7 6 5 4 3 2 1

Note: The information in this book is true and complete to the best of our knowledge. This book is intended only as an informative guide for those wishing to know more about health issues. In no way is this book intended to replace, countermand, or conflict with the advice given to you by your own physician. The ultimate decision concerning care should be made between you and your doctor. We strongly recommend you follow his or her advice. Information in this book is general and is offered with no guarantees on the part of the authors or Da Capo Press. The authors and publisher disclaim all liability in connection with the use of this book. The names and identifying details of people associated with events described in this book have been changed. Any similarity to actual persons is coincidental.

Dedicated to my parents, Gary and Harriet;
my wife, Leslie;
and my children, Shannon and Stefan
—S.H.

Dedicated to my mother, who has given me everything
—E.J.

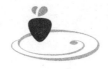

contents

introduction

YOU'RE READING THIS BOOK FOR ONE OF TWO reasons: either you want to lose weight or you just really like smoothies. We hope it is at least a little of both.

We pulled together this collection of smoothie recipes with you in mind. Yes, you. Whether you want to lose weight, maintain your current weight or gain weight, there's a smoothie for everyone. Most of our smoothies are designed to help you lose weight, but if you want to gain you can still use our recipes. You'll just have to substitute full fat ingredients for low-fat ingredients. Or add protein powder.

The point is, it is never a bad idea to put healthy things in your body. It is never a bad idea to get your full servings of fruits and vegetables every day. Smoothies help you do that, and more. But more on that in a minute.

Skinny Smoothies is not just your typical "diet" book. We're not recommending a radical program that includes deprivation and starvation. We're not advising you to drink *only* smoothies. We're recommending a lifestyle change that you can stick with for the rest of your life. We're advising you to change the way you look at food, but instead of just telling you to "eat to live" we're showing you how without sacrificing taste.

The lifestyle change is not only about smoothies. It's not just about eating foods that promote healthy detoxification of your body. It's about paying attention to the nutrients your body should receive every day, exercising regularly, and taking care of yourself the way you were intended to take care of yourself. It's simple, really. Here you'll learn how to do just that, and how to have fun with it.

About the Web site: SmoothieWeb.com

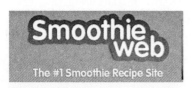

This book's genesis can be found at SmoothieWeb.com. A simple site with a simple mission: share the wonderful news of the humble smoothie. SmoothieWeb.com began one hot August night in 2006, with nothing in mind other than collecting some great recipes. The site launched with little fanfare, but since then it has grown to be the largest and most visited smoothie recipe site on earth. We hope this book provides many useful recipes, but if you are looking for even more recipes, or a few that aren't so healthy, come and visit along with the other 2.3 million smoothie lovers who visit each year.

If you stop by, please say hello and comment on our recipes. We love feedback on our smoothie recipes and look forward to receiving submissions from our fans, both new and old. In addition to the Web site we have a thriving Facebook fan page at Facebook.com/smoothieweb, and you can follow us on twitter at Twitter.com/smoothieweb. We look forward to seeing you and adding you to our smoothie family.

How to Use This Book

Before you get started making smoothies, we encourage you to read the first three chapters, which discuss detoxing, ingredients, and equipment. It's important to understand the health benefits of certain ingredients so you know (1) that you're doing something good for yourself and (2) where to fill in nutrient-wise for the rest of your day. That's what the detox chapter is for–to give you some tips on how to figure out what your daily nutrient intake should be and how to fill in the gaps on a normal week. Ultimately, there is a recipe in this book for almost every nutrient need. The nutritional information is provided to help you choose a smoothie based on what your body needs today. The recipes are just one part of your health journey. It is important to know what your body requires so that you can choose the correct smoothies to supplement your diet. Even if you're not dieting, we have smoothies to give you a burst of energy, smoothies to boost your potassium, and more.

That's the beauty of this book that bears repeating: these smoothies are great if you want to lose weight or purge toxins from your body. They're equally as great when you're healthy, happy, and at your goal weight. They're just plain good for you.

So, by all means, use this book for help making delicious, healthy smoothies so you can lose weight. But once you've lost the weight, don't pack us away. These smoothies are good every day.

Enjoy. From our blender to yours.

PART
ONE
getting started!

Health Benefits of Smoothies

About the Research

We did a lot of research on food—how it behaves in your body, what it does for your body, and how it interacts with other food. We used multiple sources and years of combined knowledge to pull together the information for the ingredients portion of Chapter 3 because we wanted to give you a strong foundation to build on. If you know the health benefits of each fruit, vegetable, and base you can get creative. So after you try each of our 101 recipes you might get adventurous and tinker with them. Tinkering is fun.

We also drew on years of combined knowledge and experimentation for the information about detoxing in this chapter. Too many deprivation diets with unsatisfactory results led us to smoothies in the first place, and we wanted to give you the benefit of our experience without you having to suffer through your first, or fifth, diet.

For the nutritional analysis we used a handy tool that is available online for free. There are lots of those out there, but we used caloriecount.about.com for consistency and because it gave us the vitamin A, vitamin C, calcium, potassium, and iron counts. We urge you to pay close attention to the nutritional information for each recipe—not just because it took us forever to compile it, but because every person is different and has different nutritional needs.

In fact, we strongly urge you to talk to your doctor before you make any drastic diet or lifestyle changes. That's just good common sense.

Toxins build up in the human body, causing the body to malfunction. If you've noticed your skin breaking out more than usual, an increase in the frequency of heartburn, or if you're feeling tired and sluggish, it could be because you have an overload of toxins in your body. Of course, any new health symptom should be discussed with your doctor, but as more doctors are aware of how diet affects the body, they might suggest that you clean up the way you eat. In a word, maybe it's time to detox.[1]

---

[1] If you are pregnant or breastfeeding, you should follow the nutritional plan outlined by your doctor. If you are under eighteen, over sixty-five, ill or recovering from being ill, or if you are taking any kind of medication, talk your detox plan over with your doctor before you begin.

A Word of Warning

The bottom line is that the fewer toxins you consume, the fewer toxins enter your body. Furthermore, the more "good" foods and beverages you consume, the easier it is for your body to get rid of toxins. There are so many "cleansing" and "detox" diets out there that is hard to know what is healthy and safe and what is dangerous.

Any diet based on deprivation is dangerous. Not only are you depriving your body of essential nutrients, but you're setting yourself up to fail. A diet where you only drink water mixed with maple syrup, lemon, and cayenne pepper might make you lose weight, but the minute you start eating normally, the weight will come back and you will most likely gain even more. Your body requires a certain amount of sustenance each day, so fasting diets are not a smart way to detox.

A diet that wants you to go to extreme measures to detox is dangerous. A plan that requires you to take a lot of fiber pills, for instance, is bad because your body must adjust to absorbing large amounts of fiber. If you overload your unprepared body with fiber you can become bloated, sick, and miserable. Additionally, any plan that wants you to administer frequent enemas is a bad plan. You need to allow your body to detoxify and eliminate naturally. Too many enemas can result in the body becoming dependent on them for evacuation, landing you in a leakier boat than you started in.

As with most things, moderation is key.

How Do You Know
If You're in Toxic Overload Mode?

The human body can acquire toxins in many ways. Toxins enter our bodies through what we eat, what we drink, environmental factors, and even from other people. The air is polluted, the water is polluted, and we consume more and more processed and refined foods every day. This gives our bodies a host of problems, all because of the toxins we absorb, and then have a hard time releasing.

A healthy body with a fully functioning immune system can usually deal with these toxins, but sometimes people aren't able to eliminate the toxins their bodies accumulate at a fast enough rate to prevent an unhealthy level of toxicity. We take in more toxins than we can eliminate, resulting in toxic bodies that can't fight off illness and infection the way they should. That's why a detoxification plan is a good idea. Some signs that you might be in toxic overload are:

- Splotchy skin or an increase in blemishes

- Frequent headaches

- Joint pain

- Nasal congestion

- Constipation

- Gas

- Heartburn

- Low energy

- Pain in the joints

- Frequent fungal infections like athlete's foot, yeast infections, etc.

- Frequent insomnia

Some of these signs can be symptoms of more serious illnesses, so if you have any doubt, see your doctor immediately. If you have a clean bill of health, yet have these persisting complaints, your body is likely loaded down with toxins and failing to function as well as it could. Some things that can cause toxic overload are:

TOBACCO: one of the worst things you can do is smoke, dip, or consume tobacco in any way whatsoever. Tobacco is loaded with carcinogens via the pesticides used on the crops and the processes used in cigarette and cigar manufacturing plants. If you are a tobacco user, your body is toxic. There are many resources available to help you quit, which is one of the hardest things you'll ever have to do. It is worth it, however, so do it.

ALCOHOL: alcohol, technically, is poison to the human body. It contains ether, which is lethal in large doses. Alcohol is also loaded with sugar. While an occasional glass of red wine can be beneficial in that it contains antioxidants and can encourage heart health, it is best to avoid alcohol on a regular basis.

PROCESSED FOODS: any processed, fried, or convenience food is likely bad for you. Stay away from additives, and you will avoid many toxins.

CAFFEINE: Caffeine is a diuretic, which means that it encourages your body to expel water. This can be good in the case of natural diuretics used to combat water weight or bloating, but caffeine is a diuretic in the worst way. It stresses your body and prevents it from absorbing key nutrients, certain vitamins, and minerals, while dehydrating it along the way.

DAIRY PRODUCTS: cow's milk makes the body produce more mucus, and many people have difficulty digesting lactose, which can cause trouble in the digestive tract.

MEAT: certain types of meat are more harmful than others. Meat that comes from animals with four legs usually contains more saturated fat, which lingers in the system as a toxin. Oily fish are your best bet for meat, though poultry once or twice a week (as long as it is organic, free range, and antibiotic-free) is okay.

WHEAT: for some people, wheat products are catastrophic. For everyone, wheat presents a certain challenge to the digestive system and can cause diarrhea, constipation, and bloating. You can get tested to see if you have intolerance to gluten, a protein composite found in wheat, rye, and barley. If you do, stay away.

REFINED SUGAR: Refined sugar has been stripped of all minerals, vitamins, and nutrients so that it is pure, refined carbohydrate. The body doesn't use refined starches unless it has the tools to help it—namely those vitamins and minerals that are stripped out of refined sugar. Because the body can't use it, refined sugar turns into pyruvic acid, which is a toxic metabolite that damages the brain and nervous system. In fact, because refined sugar is void of minerals and vitamins, it actually takes those things from the body and produces an overly acid condition in the body.

Substitutions

While many of the above items should be avoided altogether (tobacco, fried and processed food, and refined sugar), some things simply require a substitute.

Instead of consuming wheat products, try quinoa, corn, millet, buckwheat, or rice pastas. Rather than opting for a flour tortilla, choose corn, and instead of a wheat-based breakfast cereal, try oats and rye flakes. A gluten allergy can be tough, but knowing you can eat pastas and breads made out of safe items is comforting.

Rather than using refined sugar to sweeten things, try honey or organic maple syrup.

Instead of using the salt, try kicking the flavor up on your favorite dishes with fresh and dried herbs—just make sure you read labels. You can also use seaweed to get that salty taste into your food, and it is acceptable to use some salt substitutes that are herbal.

Coffee drinkers tend to believe that there is absolutely no substitute for the real thing. They are right. It takes a commitment and a lot of willpower to make the shift from coffee to herbal teas and fruit juices. It is worth it, since many teas (like green tea) can provide a dose of antioxidants, and fruit juices have many nutritional benefits, provided they are not processed and filled with sugar. (Green tea has a small amount of natural caffeine, but the health benefits outweigh the risks.) It is best to squeeze your own juices from organic fruits and vegetables—that way you know what's in there.

Instead of consuming dairy products that are cow-based, try goat's milk and cheese, soy milk products (as long as you don't have a history of breast cancer), and almond milk. If you are a fan of butter, try using hummus instead.

Detox Must-Haves

The following foods are great for someone who wants to detox.

Fruits

Apples. Apples have liver- and kidney-cleansing properties and can help extract heavy metals from the blood. They may also help lower bad cholesterol. Apples are full of fiber and also help flush the colon. An apple a day does, as it turns out, keep the doctor away.

Cranberries. Cranberries kill bacteria in the urinary tract, bladder, and kidneys. Additionally, their astringent properties help the body to expel toxins via the bowels in addition to the kidneys.

Lemons. Lemons help to detoxify the liver, and they have antibiotic properties. Additionally, citrus fruits (especially lemons and limes) can help facilitate better cell function.

Tomatoes. Tomatoes are full of lycopene, an antioxidant that helps fight cancer. Lycopene also works to protect the liver from damage done by free radicals, allowing the liver to metabolize toxins properly and eliminate them from your system.

Vegetables

Artichokes. Artichokes are a diuretic that also helps purify the liver. They contain the flavonoid silymarin, which scrubs free radicals out of the liver and helps boost liver function. Artichokes also contain cynarin, an acid found in the leaves that stimulates the liver's production of bile, which in turn helps the liver to break down fat.

Asparagus. Asparagus can preserve the "good" bacteria in the digestive tract. It's a diuretic, which flushes the system and promotes the release of toxins, and it contains fiber, which helps clean the digestive tract.

Beets. Beets contain betaine. This promotes liver cell regeneration and helps the bile to flow more freely. When that happens it helps the liver metabolize fat.

Broccoli. Broccoli is full of glutathione, which helps expel toxins from the liver by supporting enzymes in the liver that promote detoxification. Broccoli is a member of the brassica family, which also includes kale, Brussels sprouts, cabbage, and cauliflower; all are fantastic detox foods.

Carrots. Carrots are full of beta-carotene, which serves as an antibacterial and antifungal agent. They also are high in fiber, which helps the digestive tract to slough off toxins.

Fennel. Fennel is a member of the same family of vegetables as carrots, so they have similar properties, as well as containing properties that regulate contractions in the small intestine. Fennel is very calming to the digestive system, helping to relieve complications such as bloating, gas, and heartburn.

Onion. Onions contain quercetin, an antioxidant that protects the body from free radicals and encourages healthy flora in the digestive system. Flora, friendly bacteria, lives in the digestive tract and is useful in keeping you healthy. Onions are also antiviral and rich in compounds that contain sulfur. Onions and garlic both clear the detoxification pathway for the elimination of food additives and other chemicals and help the body to expel heavy metals.

Salad Greens. Salad greens clean the digestive tract because they are packed with fiber and contain antioxidants that help the body rid itself of free radicals.

Watercress. Watercress is a blood purifier, and it helps the body to expel waste by stimulating liver enzymes that promote cleansing.

Herbs and Seasonings, and Other Ingredients

Garlic. Garlic helps the body expel toxic microorganisms and provides a clear path for the liver to expel toxins (see onion for more information).

Ginger. Ginger aids in digestion and relieves stomach discomfort. It stimulates the digestive enzymes, relieving nausea, bloating, heartburn, and diarrhea.

Olive Oil. Olive oil keeps the cholesterol in food from turning into free radicals in the body. It is also full of "good" fat that is heart-healthy. Olive oil contains oleic acid, palmitic acid, and fatty acid, all of which help cleanse the gall bladder and liver.

Quinoa. An ancient grain, quinoa helps cleanse the digestive system because of the dietary fiber it contains. It is a known superfood, and it is said one could live on it alone (though we like a bit more variety).

Rice. Brown rice helps stimulate the digestive system and cleanse the colon as the rice passes through. Brown rice is said to be antiallergenic and can help to control allergic symptoms and reactions and is said to regulate blood sugar levels.

Seaweed. Seaweed helps to make the blood more alkaline and strengthens the digestive tract. Seaweed is high in iodine and is said to be an immune system booster and something that helps improve liver and thyroid function.

Yogurt. Yogurt contains live probiotics to prevent fungal infections. Also, the probiotics eliminate harmful bacteria in the wall of the intestines, resulting in the reduction of inflammation in the intestines.

Getting Ready to Detox

As you prepare to detox your body, make sure you have your kitchen stocked with the above healthy foods (as well as a selection from the foods mentioned in Chapter 3), that you have plenty of containers to store fresh fruits and vegetables, and that you have the proper equipment for juicing, making smoothies, and drying fruit, if necessary. Please refer to Chapter 3 for more information on choosing the right equipment.

Start weaning yourself off the things you consume that promote toxicity in your body. Shock to the digestive system can be harmful, so easing yourself into a detoxifying diet is better than starting gung-ho after no preparation whatsoever. Moderation is key.

Make sure you have a source for plenty of clean, filtered, pure water. Water is the most important component of any successful detox plan.

Have a way to reward yourself for your good work that does not include introducing more toxins into your system. A massage, while releasing toxins into your bloodstream, will ultimately allow you to eliminate those toxins, provided you are eating healthy, detoxifying food and exercising regularly. Also, yoga can be quite rewarding and will help you dispel other types of toxins, like emotional and spiritual woes. If you need an even bigger treat, think about a new outfit for your slimming body, a new pair of exercise shoes, or even a new hairdo. You deserve it.

Throw out any foods, beverages, or substances that will hinder your detoxification efforts. It is hard to eat the potato chips if they are not in your house.

Ultimately, pace yourself and be kind to your body.

What to Expect from Detox

First and foremost, you can expect, from following a detoxification program, to lose weight in a healthy way, to shed your body of toxins that impede good health, and to feel great about yourself. But it takes some time to get there. People have varying levels of toxicity in their bodies, depending on their age, lifestyle, and food choices. Detoxing can take a long time, especially if you do it correctly with life changes, rather than crash diets or deprivation detox plans. Some temporary things you might experience as a result of your body's release of long-lingering toxins are an increase in acne or skin blemishes; digestive upset in the form of diarrhea, heartburn, gas, or bloating; and feeling tired and grouchy as your body adjusts to this new way of living. Be patient and don't give up, but if you have health issues that concern you, it is best to see your family doctor to be sure that you are helping your body, not hurting it.

After you've followed a clean diet and have implemented an exercise program, not only can you expect to feel better and be thinner, but you can expect your hair and skin to be healthier, and your mind as well. Here's to a healthier new you!

2

Your Daily Intake

EACH OF THE SMOOTHIES in this sample section replaces a meal, but none of them provides all the nutrients you need for a balanced diet. You should be consuming lean protein, whole grains, and vegetables as part of your weight loss or detox program. To make sure you're getting the right amount of calories, carbohydrates, protein, fiber, and more, follow some simple guidelines. There are lots of free tools online that will help you calculate your daily intake. For example, if you are a mildly active forty-five-year-old woman who is about 5'5" and weighs about 150 pounds, some of your nutritional requirements will differ from a twenty-five-year-old man who is very active, 6'2," and weighs 210 pounds. See the difference in the chart below.

| | SAMPLE | |
	Woman	Man
Calories	1200	2,105
Carbohydrates	150 g	263 g
Fat	40 g	70 g
Saturated Fat	4 g	7 g
Protein	60 g	105 g
Fiber	25 g	25 g
Sugar	64 g	64 g
Sodium	2,400 mg	2,400 mg
Cholesterol	300 mg	300 mg
Vitamin A	5,000 IU	5,000 IU
Vitamin C	60 mg	60 mg
Iron	18 mg	18 mg
Calcium	1,000 mg	1,000 mg
Potassium	3,500 mg	3,500 mg

Source: http://www.dietitian.com/

The Sugar Question

You might notice that the sugar recorded in each nutritional analysis seems high. Fresh fruits do contain sugar, but they contain simple sugar—fructose—that the body can metabolize quickly, meaning that the sugar doesn't hang around long enough to convert to fat in your body (as long as you're active).

The dangerous type of sugar—refined sugar—is the thing you should be looking out for. Colas and sodas, sweets, items made from white flour, fried food, and even energy bars contain refined sugar and complex carbohydrates, which the body stores and then converts to fat.

The Sample Week

Risking repetition, detoxifying your body is not the same thing as a cleanse. In a cleanse you would drink the smoothies below and consume only fruits, vegetables, and a bit of vegetable broth. To us, detoxing is a way of life—it's about putting healthy things into your body that nourish and sustain you while allowing you to lose weight and drive out the toxins. The sample week that follows is an example of how you should eat all the time, perhaps eventually substituting the detox smoothies for other healthy smoothies depending on your body's needs.

Day 1

To start purifying your body, try the **Fruity Dandelion Smoothie** (page 182) first thing in the morning, followed by plenty of water. Midmorning, grab a piece of fruit full of water, like watermelon, accompanied by some skim dairy, like a piece of low-fat string cheese.

For lunch, have lean protein like low-fat, low-sodium turkey on a piece of whole-grain bread, and a serving of vegetables—preferably leafy greens.

For an afternoon snack have a vegetable, for example, some carrots or celery sticks.

For dinner, have more lean protein like grilled chicken with fresh herbs (a serving no larger than the palm of your hand) and plenty of vegetables like broccoli, Brussels sprouts, or some other cruciferous veggie.

For the rest of the week, follow the same instructions for your midmorning snack, lunch, afternoon snack, and dinner. Make sure you get all the nutrients you need for a balanced meal. Drinking smoothies that aren't high in calories but high in protein are best for lunch and snacks.

Other examples of good proteins are: white meat turkey, salmon, tuna, egg whites, beans, nuts, soy, and quinoa (which has the added benefit of being a grain with lots of fiber).

Examples of grains are quinoa (mentioned above), barley, bulgur, flaxseed, wild rice, brown rice, oats, rye, and spelt.

Day 2

Continue to detoxify your body with the **Classic Green Detox Smoothie** (page 143) and plenty of water, plus the dietary guidelines outlined above.

Day 3

Keep on your detox plan with the **Simple Smoothie Detox** (page 145). The tang from the grapefruit will give you a great start for your day.

Day 4

Start your day with the **Merry Morning Smoothie** (page 72), moving out of the detox smoothies and into the weight loss smoothies.

Day 5

Start off with the **Ruby Red Smoothie** (page 79) for a great boost of fiber and a more robust smoothie.

Day 6

Kick start your day with lots of antioxidants and nutrients with the **Cherry Buzz** (page 115).

Day 7

Fiber, protein, and healthy fat—that's what you'll get with the **Power Strawberry Smoothie** (page 99).

3

Ingredients and Equipment

Equipment

One of the wonderful things about smoothies—besides their obvious health benefits and delicious flavors—is how simple they are to make. Very few kitchen items other than a blender are needed. And most of the equipment you will need you most likely already own. Here are the kitchen items we recommend.

The Blender

This will be the most expensive piece of equipment you will need to buy and is a worthwhile investment for your kitchen. While just about any blender will mix or blend your ingredients into a smoothie, there are some very important things to consider when choosing your blender. Making an informed choice in the beginning will give you the best results long-term and save you some frustration.

The best blenders are from Blendtec and Vitamix. They build and sell excellent blenders and if you have the budget to afford a blender from either company, you cannot go wrong. A quality blender from Vitamix or Blendtec can easily cost several hundred dollars, so if this is beyond your budget the good news is you can find an acceptable blender to get you started for much less.

There are certainly blenders that you can buy that are very inexpensive (cheap) for around $50, but you will find yourself replacing these blenders often, cleaning up messes and drinking poorly mixed smoothies. These cheap blenders wear out quickly and will struggle to make many smoothies in this book, particularly when ice is involved.

Blenders in the midrange price of $75–$130 are going to be a better investment for your dollar. They have many of the characteristics you will require for making better smoothies. Blenders in this price range will provide most of the basics for making smoothies until you are ready for a top-of-the-line blender.

As we mentioned, Vitamix and Blendtec are the leaders in blender manufacturing; their blenders are built for commercial use. These machines will easily handle any smoothie recipe you can throw at them. These blenders will last for years, come with long warranties, and are meant for daily use. A blender you buy from Vitamix and Blendtec could easily be the last blender you buy.

Regardless of your price range, there are some characteristics your blender should have:

- **Base:** For stability, the blender should be heavy with a sturdy base, preferably made with metal.

- **Motor:** The motor should be at least 350–500 watts. This is a minimum and the more you can afford the better. Higher watts means more power for pureeing frozen fruits, frozen vegetables, and ice.

- **Speed Control:** A variable speed control is helpful as it gives you the ability to slowly increase your blade speed. We like a dial for maximum control, but at least three speeds should be available.

- **Carafe:** Your carafe (jug or pitcher) should be made from glass or a polycarbonate plastic. Many people would suggest glass over polycarbonate plastic, but for safety reasons we prefer polycarbonate plastic. The carafe should be square not circular; this provides better blending of ingredients.

- **Lids:** Lids should be heavy and fit firmly in the carafe's opening. Loose-fitting lids that don't secure tightly will lead to cleanups. You don't want to clean liquefied blueberry from your ceiling.

- **Blade Assembly:** This should be fixed to the carafe. Cleanup may not be as easy, but leaks are worse. The interlocking gears should be made of metal, not plastic.

- **Accessories:** A blender plunger can be your best friend and higher-end blenders come with one. You can use a wooden spoon, but be ready to buy a lot of wooden spoons. Never, ever use your fingers—they are much harder to replace.

What blender do we recommend? The Vitamix Super 5200 makes incredible smoothies and sounds like an airplane taking off with its 2-peak HP (1380 Watts) motor. We have yet to see it struggle with any smoothie recipe. This is a blender you have for a lifetime and then hand down to your children. We recommend it on Smoothieweb.com as our blender of choice (http://www.smoothieweb.com/smoothie -store/).

Knives

Don't try to save money on knives. As with a blender, buy the best you can afford. Choose heavy knives that are well balanced. The following knives will be useful for preparing your smoothie ingredients.

- **Chef's knife**—a good all-purpose knife, 8–10 inches in length, is ideal for cutting fruits and vegetables as well as chopping herbs.

- **Utility knife**—useful for light chopping and slicing, usually about 5–7 inches in length.

- **Paring knife**—perfect for peeling fruits and vegetables and chopping small items.

Chopping Boards

Keep a separate chopping board for your fruits and vegetables. Never use it to chop meat, poultry, or fish, which will prevent cross-contamination. Wood or polyethylene boards are both good choices for chopping fruits and vegetables. Wood cannot be sterilized but if you are only chopping fruits and vegetables on it you should be fine. Polyethylene boards can be sterilized and are dishwasher safe.

Grater

A standard grater will be fine for smoothie recipes. It should be able to grate your citrus rinds and ginger root.

Corer

Corers provide a clean, cylindrical cut. You can also cut the fruit in pieces that need coring and then use a paring knife to remove the core.

Peelers

The most popular peelers fall into a few categories and are a matter of preference.

- **Y-shaped peelers**—ideal for thick-skinned vegetables

- **Lancashire peeler**—recommended for thick-skinned fruits and vegetables

- **Australian peeler**—distinguished by a partially rotating blade that makes it easier and quicker to peel vegetables

Ingredients

The taste, texture, and health benefits of your smoothie will depend on the ingredients you use. You may have made smoothies in the past using the tastiest ingredients you could find, knowing nothing about the health benefits or risks of what you put in the blender. That's where a handy ingredient dictionary can help—after reading this chapter you will know the benefits of the fruits, vegetables, herbs, liquids, and ingredients we suggest in our recipes. And while not all the ingredients we list here are used in the collected smoothies, you will have a better understanding of when you want to use the ingredients as you continue to make your own healthy recipes.

You'll find this ingredients list divided into sections. This will make it easier to look up a specific ingredient by food type. We'll start with the fruits, then vegetables, herbs and supplements, and finally the liquids that make up the ingredients in our smoothie recipes. Each section will have the ingredients listed alphabetically so they're easy to find. Please note that ingredients with detox properties are marked by an asterisk (*).

Fruits

A

Acai.* The acai berry has a rich, chocolaty taste and is a great fruit for bulking up the texture of your smoothie. Other than that, it is a powerful antioxidant and may have anticancer properties. It is high in fiber, omega-6 and omega-9 fatty acids, potassium, zinc, and magnesium. You can buy acai berries frozen at many natural foods stores.

Apple.* An apple a day truly can help keep the doctor away. Apples not only taste good, but they act as a digestive diuretic and a liver stimulant, and they help to lower blood cholesterol. Apples contain vitamin A, vitamin C, vitamin B, and riboflavin and have been used in some countries to treat urinary tract disorders, rheumatism, and gout. Sometimes, smoothie recipes call for apple juice instead of actual apples—in these instances it is best to juice your own apples, since apple juices that can be bought at stores are often full of high-fructose corn syrup and other added ingredients.

Apricot. Apricots are loaded with beta-carotene, which can help break down cholesterol in the body. This helps keep the heart healthy. Apricots are high in potassium, boron, magnesium, vitamin B_2, and fiber. They are great additions to smoothies, especially in their dried form, because they add sweetness.

Avocado. Avocados, usually mistaken as part of the vegetable group, are fruits with high concentrations of potassium (second only to bananas) and essential fatty acids. Avocados are full of protein and contain vitamin A, vitamin C, vitamin E, each B vitamin except for B_{12}, iron, magnesium, niacin, and calcium. This creamy fruit has high oil content, so small amounts of avocado in your smoothie recipe are best, lest your smoothie have an oily texture. Avocados are seasonal, but because they are so popular, you can find them imported in almost any grocery store. It is best to buy organic.

B

Banana. Bananas are smoothie superstars. They add a wonderful thick and creamy texture to a smoothie along with their distinctive, fruity flavor. They provide an antibacterial service to the body and help the body fight ulcers by strengthening the walls of the lining of the stomach. They help boost the body's immune system and can help lower cholesterol in the blood. Bananas hold the distinction of being the fruit with the highest level of potassium.

Blackberry. Blackberries have antioxidant properties and contain vitamin C, potassium, calcium, and iron, as well as fiber. They are seasonal, but readily available frozen and canned in the off months. If you buy fresh blackberries to use in a smoothie, use them right away, because (even refrigerated) they spoil very easily. If you buy frozen black-berries, opt for the organic type.

Black Currant.* Black currants are not only antioxidants but also have anticancer, antibacterial, and antidiarrheal properties and can boost the immune system to fight infection and accelerate the healing process. That's a good fruit! Unfortunately, they are not available at every common grocery store, but some of the health food and organic stores carry them either fresh (more rare), or frozen. They are also available dried, but whole currants with the seeds provide the most health benefit.

Blueberry.* Blueberries are antiviral, antibacterial, antidiarrheal, and loaded with antioxidants. They contain tannins, which provide antibacterial and antiviral proper-ties, and are high in vitamin C, fiber, and potassium. Fresh blueberries make the best smoothies but can be expensive. If you opt for frozen blueberries, just make sure you choose the organic brands, available in most grocery stores. Wild blueberries offer a slightly different taste and are somewhat smaller, but every bit as healthy.

C

Cantaloupe.* Cantaloupes have antioxidant properties in their effective use of vitamin A. The cantaloupe is high in beta-carotene, which converts to vitamin A inside the body. This can promote lung health. Cantaloupes are also high in vitamin C, vitamin E, and fiber. Cantaloupe provides a refreshing change from your standard strawberry or banana smoothies—just make sure you use fresh cantaloupe for the correct taste and consistency. Cantaloupe is seasonal, so enjoy it while you can!

Cherry.* Not only are cherries delicious, they are also anti-bacterial, anticancer, and act as an antioxidant in the body. The ellagic acid present in cherries is what makes them such great cancer fighters, and the tiny fruits are also full of vitamin A, potassium, and vitamin C. Cherries add great flavor to a smoothie, and black cherries have the added benefit of being good for the teeth. If fresh cherries are out of season, dried cherries, frozen cherries, or canned cherries will work—just make sure you remove any pits!

Citrus Fruit.* Oranges, grapefruits, lemons, limes, tangerines, and clementines are all citrus fruit, and they all contain antioxidants and some cancer-fighting properties. All citrus fruit is packed with vitamin C and high in limonene. Some studies have shown that limonene is effective in the inhibition of breast cancer cells. As for the individual fruits—they have some magic powers of their own:

Lemon—helps detoxify the liver and facilitates better cell function

Lime—helps with cell function

Orange—contains choline, a substance that helps the brain

Red grapefruit—high in lycopene, a known cancer fighter

Try to buy organic whenever possible—nonorganic companies tend to inject gas into citrus fruits to make them retain their shape and color. When making a smoothie with the juice of a citrus fruit, take the time to juice the fruit yourself, so that you can reap the wonderful health benefits of citrus.

Coconut. Coconut is high in fiber and possesses antiviral properties. The flesh of the coconut is not used in smoothies as often as coconut milk is—see the section on Liquids and Bases (page 62) for more information.

Cranberry.* Cranberries kill bacteria in the urinary tract, bladder, and kidneys, and their astringent properties help the body to expel toxins through the bowels. Cranberries are antiviral, antibacterial, anticancer, and antioxidant. They are high in vitamin A, vitamin C, calcium, and iodine. Cranberries have an extremely tart taste, so make sure your other smoothie ingredients work to counter that tart taste—unless, of course, you like it! Fresh cranberries are best for smoothies, though you can use store-bought cranberry juice as long as you are sure that cranberries are the only ingredient. As with most fruits added to smoothies, freezing the fruit for later use is a great option. You can freeze cranberries for later use since finding fresh cranberries year-round can be difficult.

D

Date.* Dates stimulate the colon and act as a laxative in the system. They are also shown to boost estrogen levels, so if you have a personal history of breast cancer, it is best to avoid them. People with a history of migraine headaches would probably do best to avoid dates as well, unless they are sure that dates are not a headache trigger. Dates prevent calcium loss because they contain boron, and they contain vitamin A, C, D, B_1, and B_2. Dates will thicken and sweeten a smoothie. They are seasonal, and can be found at Middle Eastern grocery stores.

F

Fig.* Figs are antibacterial, antiulcer, anticancer, and stimulate the colon, acting as a laxative. Their cancer-fighting agent is benzaldehyde, and they are high in potassium and calcium. Like dates, figs can be a headache trigger for some people, so if you are one of them, leave them out of your smoothie. Figs are seasonal, like dates, and can be found in Middle Eastern grocery stores. You can use fresh figs or dried figs (available year-round).

G

Grape.* Grapes are high in ellagic acid and caffeic acids, which are anticancer agents. Grapes are also antiviral and antioxidant. Grapes are high in flavonoids, which are heart-healthy, and they contain boron, which helps the body retain calcium. Make sure you buy organic grapes—nonorganic grapes are known to be full of pesticides. For your smoothie, use seedless grapes.

H

Honeydew. Honeydew melons contain antioxidants and also have anticoagulant properties because they contain adenosine. This helps reduce the risk of stroke and heart attack. They are a great source of vitamin A and C, and they add a sweet taste to a smoothie. Just add some peeled chunks of honeydew to your smoothie for a special, fresh treat.

K

Kiwifruit.* Kiwi aids in digestion and also is high in vitamin C. Kiwifruit is special because it actually contains vitamin E. The antioxidants in kiwi help to protect the body's cells from free-radical damage. Many people use kiwi as part of a detox plan, because of the way it aids the body's digestion. Use fresh kiwi in your smoothie for a digestive boost that tastes great.

M

Mango.* High in beta-carotene (and therefore vitamin A), mangoes are antioxidant and anticancer, and they help protect the arteries from blockage. Also high in fiber, mangoes help the body eliminate, and they may also help fight infection. Make sure every bit of the skin is removed, as the sap within it is known to cause irritation and cube the fresh mango for use in a smoothie to give it that boost of vitamin A and a nice, creamy texture.

N

Nectarine.* Nectarines possess antioxidant and anticancer properties because they are a great source of potassium and vitamins A and C. They are an ancient fruit and are a cultivar form of peaches. Nectarines can even bud from peach trees. They add sweetness and plenty of health benefits to smoothies. Remove the pit and add to the blender with the skin on.

P

Papaya.* Papayas have many beneficial properties. They possess antioxidants and anticancer properties because of their high concentration of vitamins A and C and can aid digestion. Papayas are sweet and add a creamy texture to your smoothie. Just make sure you use the seeds, since they are full of protein.

Peach. Peaches have niacin, vitamin A, and potassium, as well as anticancer and antioxidant properties. For a fruit, they are surprisingly low in sugar and are thought to prevent cancer, heart disease, and osteoporosis. When you can use fresh peaches, remove the pit and skin and use the tasty, sweet flesh to add texture and flavor to your smoothies. When peaches are out of season, use canned peaches, which offer almost all of the same benefits as fresh peaches.

Pear.* Pears are high in fiber and help build up the walls of the digestive system, especially the colon. They are great for detoxing and are a source of potassium, boron, and vitamin C. If the pears are organic, it is fine to use the peel, and you'll get extra fiber that way. If they are not organic, peel fresh pears before adding them to your smoothie. When pears are not in season, you can use frozen or canned pears. Be sure you check the ingredients to make sure there is no sugar added.

Pineapple. Pineapples are packed with potassium and, despite their acidity, can help aid digestion. Since fresh pineapple is so hard to work with, it is fine to use canned pineapple or frozen pineapple, just make sure it is free of added sugar.

Plum.* Plums have antibacterial and antioxidant properties, mainly because they are a source of vitamin A. They also boast calcium and a smidge of vitamin C. Plums (the fresh source of prunes) can provide relief to constipation, so if you're using them for detox purposes, use the prune form of the fruit.

Pomegranate. Pomegranate seeds are actually shown to reduce fevers! So, next time you have a nasty fever, throw together a smoothie that contains pomegranates. They are also astringent to the system and have antioxidant properties. They contain flavonoids and tannins to help fight cancer, and you can throw the seeds in your smoothie for all the benefits, including fiber.

R

Raspberry. Raspberries boost the immune system, making them not only tasty, but super healthy. They contain potassium and niacin, which helps reduce cholesterol in the blood. Raspberries have to be used soon after buying, so you might want to opt for organic frozen raspberries. They add a sweet, fresh taste to smoothies.

S

Strawberry.* Strawberries have so many health benefits, they are a superfood. They are antiviral and possess antioxidant properties. They contain ellagic acid, a cancer fighter, and they help treat gout, rheumatism, and kidney stones. They provide cleansing actions on the liver and can be used for cleansing as they help with elimination. They work in almost every smoothie recipe, and you can use organic frozen strawberries if fresh ones aren't in season.

W

Watermelon.* In addition to being very tasty, watermelon has high water content, so it is great for early-morning smoothies when you're trying to consume mainly water-based foods. Watermelon is antibacterial and can fight cancer because of its high concentration of vitamin A; it is also high in vitamin C and iron.

Vegetables

A

Artichoke. Artichokes possess antibacterial properties, and contain iron, calcium, and magnesium. To use a fresh artichoke heart in a smoothie, blanch it first and let it cool, then chop it and put it into your smoothie mixture.

Arugula.* Arugula is not only a tasty green; it is also very good for you. Full of fiber, vitamins C, A, K, and P, potassium, and iron, it helps cleanse the blood, which in turn helps cleanse the liver. Throw a handful into a tomato-based smoothie for an extra kick of health.

Asparagus.* Asparagus provides a load of health benefits—it can help prevent cataracts, is a diuretic, contains antioxidants, fights off cancer, and can help the body heal faster. Asparagus contains vitamin C, vitamin A, and the elusive vitamin E. Boil for a few minutes and let cool before adding asparagus to your smoothie.

B

Bean.* Italian green beans, string beans, wax beans, kidney beans, pintos, and snow peas—they are full of antioxidants and are thought to help improve memory function. Dried beans, when available, have more nutrients than fresh beans, so for smoothies go ahead and soak overnight, shell, and then add to a smoothie for added protein and thickness. If using green beans, opt for fresh instead of canned.

Beet.* Beets contain betaine, an enzyme that does wonders for the gallbladder and liver. They are also antibacterial, contain antioxidants, and can provide cleansing properties. You can use any sort of cooked beets in your smoothie—if fresh ones aren't in season, use canned or frozen for a punch of cleansing power.

Bell Pepper. Green, orange, red, and yellow bell peppers have antioxidant properties and can help protect the heart, as well as guard against cancer. Throw them into a vegetable smoothie for great taste and heart protection.

Broccoli.* Broccoli is full of glutathione, which helps expel toxins from the liver by supporting enzymes that promote detoxification. Broccoli also contains indoles and glucosinolates that help fight cancer and is considered a superfood. It has high concentrations of vitamin A and C. You can use fresh or frozen broccoli in your smoothie, and with the right concentration of fruit, you don't even have to taste it.

C

Cabbage.* All varieties of cabbage contain antibacterial, anticancer, and antioxidant properties. Cabbage can prevent cataracts, help retain brain function, detoxify the body, and encourage healing. It contains the elusive vitamin E and is great for the liver and colon. Shred fresh cabbage into your smoothie for all these great health benefits.

Carrot.* Carrots are full of beta-carotene, which serves as an antibacterial and antifungal agent. They are also high in fiber and help the body slough off toxins. Carrots are shown to prevent constipation, can lower cholesterol, and contain antioxidants. They are, as it turns out, good for your eyes, and the cooked carrot has even more cancer-fighting power, as cooking releases the carotenes (thus releasing the vitamin A), but stem your carrots slightly before adding them to your smoothie.

Cauliflower.* Cauliflower, like broccoli, has antioxidant and anticancer properties, and it contains vitamin C. Cook it before putting in into your smoothie, lest you have an unpleasant texture in the smoothie.

Celery.* Celery is a mild diuretic and provides a detoxifying effect on the body, helping the body to rid itself of carcinogens. Throw in some raw, chopped celery for a great taste and great health benefits.

Chile Peppers.* Chiles contain capsaicin, which helps reduce inflammation in the body. Chiles are antiseptic and antibacterial and can help prevent lung disorders, act as an expectorant with bronchitis, and help thin the blood. Because of this particular property of the chile, it rates high on heart-healthy things to consume, since a veggie that can thin the blood will reduce the risk of clotting. So, if you have a clotting problem, it's best to stay away. You can use fresh, canned, or dried chile peppers in your smoothie for an extra zing and loads of health benefits.

Corn.* Corn helps the body retain a balanced pH in the stomach, because it helps to neutralize stomach acid. It is also high in fiber, so it can act as a laxative with a cleansing impact to the colon and digestive tract. Corn may also raise estrogen levels and can prevent kidney stones. Smoothies are a great way to get rid of extra cooked fresh corn—just scrape it off the cob into the blender. You can also use canned corn, just make sure you don't use creamed corn or flavored corn.

Cucumber. Cucumbers are full of water, making them a great moisture addition to your smoothie. They also contain sterols, known to lower cholesterol. Remove the skin, but leave in the seeds for the most nutritional benefit in your smoothie.

D

Dandelion Greens. Dandelion greens are high in vitamins A, C, and K and also contain plenty of iron. They contain anti-inflammatory properties and may help counter urinary tract infections because of their diuretic properties. Throw in a few handfuls for a healthy, green smoothie.

E

Eggplant. Eggplant is also a diuretic and possesses antibacterial properties. It also contains terpenes, which work against steroidal hormones that would otherwise promote cancer cells in the body. Eggplant also contains potassium, which can help lower blood pressure. Peel the eggplant and chunk it into your smoothie to add these health benefits plus fiber. Eggplant does not have a strong taste, so it will add texture to your smoothie without an overpowering flavor.

F

Fennel. Fennel is a member of the same family of vegetables as carrots, so the two have similar properties, as well as containing properties that regulate contractions in the small intestine. Fennel is calming to the digestive system, helping to relieve complications such as gas, bloating, and heartburn.

G

Garlic. Garlic has antibiotic properties, as well as antimicrobial, anticancer, antihistamine, antiparasitic, and diuretic properties. It inhibits the proliferation of cancer cells and can protect organs against damage from toxins. Use fresh cloves of garlic in your vegetable smoothie for great taste and fantastic health benefits. An added function of garlic is that it makes you unattractive to fleas, mosquitoes, and other biting insects.

K

Kale. Kale is a leafy green and contains antioxidant and anticancer properties because it is high in vitamin A, iron, folic acid, and potassium. Leave out the ribs and stems, and chop kale greens for a powerful green smoothie.

L

Leek.* Leeks pack a detox punch because the body digests them so easily. They are antiseptic and provide a laxative reaction in the body. They are also great for colds and other respiratory illnesses, as they are an expectorant. Cut off the bright green leaves and the end of the bulb, then chop the leek and wash the pieces. Dirt tends to cling on these healthy members of the onion family. Raw, they are very pungent with an onion flavor. They sweeten a little when cooked.

Lettuce. Green leafy lettuces like romaine and green leaf are high in fiber, vitamin A, iron, and folic acid and can be added to smoothies for a green, healthy smoothie.

O

Onion.* Onions contain quercetin, an antioxidant that protects the body from free radicals and encourages healthy flora in the digestive system. Onions are also antiviral and rich in compounds that contain sulfur. Onions clear the detoxification pathway for the elimination of food additives and other chemicals and help the body to expel heavy metals.

P

Potato. Potatoes contain potassium, which protects the heart. They are also high in fiber and a good source of B vitamins. The body has a hard time digesting white and red potatoes along with a protein source, so if you're looking for a potato combination with protein, opt for a gold potato. The body processes gold potatoes much more easily. If you are sticking with straight fruits and veggies for a smoothie, use whatever potato you like best.

S

Spinach.* Spinach is loaded with fiber and helps clean the digestive tract. It also contains antioxidants that help rid the digestive tract of free radicals. Buy organic spinach and throw a handful or two into your smoothie for a detoxifying effect.

Squash. Squash, as well as pumpkin, is high in vitamin A, so that means it has anticancer properties, as well as antioxidant properties. Use cooked squash for the best texture in your smoothie.

Sweet Potato. Sweet potatoes are high in fiber, beta carotene, and vitamin C and are rich in complex carbs. They have anticancer properties as well as antioxidant properties and are a good food for diabetics, because they may help stabilize blood sugar.

Swiss Chard. Swiss chard is high in vitamins C, K, and A, and it is high in dietary fiber. Add stalks and leaves to smoothies for a health boost.

T

Tomato. Tomatoes have antioxidant and anticancer properties, mainly because they are a great source of lycopene and glutathione. They also have glutamic acid. The body converts glutamic acid into gamma-aminobutryic acid, which is proven to fight kidney hypertension. Use cooked or fresh tomatoes in a smoothie for a great taste, and many health benefits.

W

Watercress. * Watercress is a blood purifier and helps the body to expel waste. Watercress possesses anticancer, diuretic, antibiotic, and antioxidant properties and helps stimulate liver enzymes that promote cleansing. This powerful green packs quite a punch so only use about three sprigs in your smoothie.

Z

Zucchini. Zucchini contains vitamin C, vitamin A, potassium, and niacin, which is proven to lower cholesterol. You can remove the skin if you aren't able to buy organic zucchini, but if the zucchini is organic or homegrown, feel free use the skin when you chop the zucchini to put it into your smoothie.

Herbs and Other Supplements

A

Alfalfa.* Alfalfa is a perennial, and it has loads of health benefits but should be used with caution. Alfalfa provides a tonic for the body, and it nourishes the cells. It supports connective tissue, teeth, and bones, and it promotes healing and may ease arthritis. However, alfalfa sprouts and seeds contain canavanine, an amino acid that, in some people, exacerbates their arthritis, instead of soothing it. Alfalfa leaves do not contain canavanine, so they are safe for inflammatory conditions.

B

Basil. Fragrant and tasty, basil can be used to fight headaches, stress, indigestion, and tension because they contain antibacterial, antidepressant, and antispasmodic properties. Basil also stimulates the adrenal gland, which contributes to its antidepressant properties. Chop off the stems and throw them away, and chop up the yummy leaves to put them in your smoothie for a refreshing taste.

Brewer's Yeast. Brewer's yeast is high in nucleic acid, which helps cells develop. It also is high in folic acid, niacin (which helps lower cholesterol), chromium (which aids the body in the production of insulin), and potassium. Brewer's yeast can also boost the metabolism, making it a power ingredient for smoothies. You can buy brewer's yeast in health stores, but remember to get the pure form, rather that the debittered, as the bitter type contains the beneficial nutrients. Just make sure you use it with a sweet or savory, strong smoothie ingredient so you don't have to taste it.

C

Cardamom.* Cardamom stimulates the digestive tract, making it a good ingredient for a detox smoothie. It also can stimulate the appetite and dispel gas. You can buy whole cardamom seeds at your local grocery store—just grind them before adding the ingredient to smoothies.

Cayenne.* Cayenne is a powerful derivative of a chile plant, so it contains capsaicin, which helps purify the blood and promote elimination. Cayenne should not be used in cases of IBS or Crohn's disease, and it should be avoided during pregnancy. You can use cayenne peppers or the dried spice in your smoothies for a kick of heat and spice.

Celery Seed.* Celery seed contains anti-inflammatory and antioxidant properties, making it a tonic that helps soothe muscle spasms, can reduce inflammation, and may be good for urinary tract infections. Avoid celery seed if you're pregnant. For smoothies, crush the seeds and use sparingly.

Chamomile. Chamomile has anti-inflammatory and antiseptic properties and has a mild sedative effect. Chamomile contains thujone, an oil that has emmenagogue properties, which means that it stimulates the uterus, so should be avoided during pregnancy. If you're not pregnant, chamomile can relieve anxiety, ease menstrual cramps, settle the stomach, and dispel gas. Use fresh petals and flowers in your smoothie.

Cider Vinegar. Cider vinegar produces an alkaline response in the body and can be used to relieve a host of ailments, including colds, allergies, stomach pains, and indigestion, and it can promote "good" bacteria. Add a teaspoon of all-natural, raw, and unfiltered apple cider vinegar to smoothies.

Cinnamon. Cinnamon is a carminative that can soothe the stomach, relieving diarrhea, nausea, and vomiting. Use ground cinnamon in your smoothie to soothe your stomach and provide that delicious, warming taste.

Clove.* Clove flowers have antioxidant, anti-inflammatory, anesthetic, and antihistamine properties. Clove has been used to treat respiratory and stomach problems, and it might have anticancer properties. Use ¼ teaspoon for smoothies.

Coriander. Coriander is wonderful for soothing digestive woes like nausea and flatulence and can stimulate the appetite. Crush dried seeds to powder and add ½ teaspoon to smoothies.

Cumin. Cumin can stimulate the colon, but it also soothes the digestive tract. It is also thought to increase milk flow in women who are breastfeeding. Crush dried seeds into a powder and add ¼ to ½ teaspoon per smoothie.

D

Dill. Dill seeds are thought to increase milk flow in women who are breastfeeding and also have antispasmodic and soothing properties. Crush dried seeds to powder and use ¼ to ½ teaspoon per smoothie.

E

Echinacea. Echinacea is known for its immune-boosting, anti-inflammatory properties. It also contains antimicrobial, antiseptic, antiallergenic, and antibiotic properties. Cook the chopped root and add to smoothies to heal anything from sinus woes to urinary tract infections.

Evening Primrose. Evening primrose oil acts as an anticoagulant that improves circulation of the blood, and contains fatty acids that help repair tissue. Evening primrose oil has been used to treat everything from acne to PMS. The easiest way to buy it is in capsules. Just split the capsule open and pour the oil into the blender before you mix your smoothie.

F

Fennel. Fennel seeds are soothing, contain anti-inflammatory and antispasmodic properties, and have also been shown to increase milk flow in breastfeeding women. The seeds are a uterine stimulant, so do not use fennel seeds if you are pregnant. Crush dried seeds to powder for smoothies.

Feverfew. Feverfew leaves have been known to help prevent migraines and can help ease rheumatoid arthritis pain and menstrual cramps. Feverfew also stimulates the uterus, so avoid it if you're pregnant, and avoid chewing fresh leaves. Use dried leaves crushed to powder in your smoothie.

Flax.* Flaxseed oil is loaded with omega-3 fatty acids, which is fabulous for the joints and skin. It helps the joints avoid absorbing toxins and stimulates digestion. You can buy flax seeds at any health food store and just add seeds to smoothies for the health boost and a smooth, nutty taste.

G

Ginger.* Ginger aids in digestion and relieves stomach discomfort. It stimulates the digestive enzymes, relieving nausea, bloating, gas, heartburn, and diarrhea. Ginger has anti-inflammatory properties, making it useful in treating symptoms associated with arthritis and headaches. It also can combat morning sickness.

Ginkgo. Ginkgo is commonly thought to help brain function, and it contains antioxidant properties, increases blood flow, and can help relieve some symptoms of bronchitis. Use ginkgo leaves, dried and ground into a powder, for your smoothies—about 1 teaspoon per smoothie.

Ginseng. Ginseng can settle the stomach, and it can regulate cholesterol and blood sugar. It has antioxidant properties and can help battle stress. Ginseng also increases energy levels, so don't use it if you are drinking coffee the same day and also avoid ginseng if you are pregnant or nursing. Use the fresh ginseng root (organic) with the skin on for the most health benefits.

Green Algae.* Green algae can help the body rid itself of heavy metals, can boost immunity, and has anticancer and antioxidant properties. Some specialists claim that green algae can counter harmful radiation effects and may be helpful in treating infections related to HIV. To add green algae to your smoothie, add 2 teaspoons of the powder.

Green Tea.* Green tea leaves have antioxidant properties but can also act as a diuretic and help prevent cancer. Additionally, some have reported that green tea, when ingested a week prior to exposure to radiation, has lessened the discomfort of treatments. Crush tea leaves into a fine powder and use a few teaspoons in your smoothie.

H

Hemp. Hemp seeds are full of omega-3 and omega-6 fatty acids, as well as being a good source of protein. Throw hulled hemp seeds (also called hemp nuts) into your smoothie for a nutty, earthy flavor and smooth texture.

Honey. Honey contains antibacterial, antimicrobial, and antioxidant properties and is also a stomach-soother. Honey is naturally sweet but contains vitamins and minerals, so the sweetness is beneficial. Add honey to any smoothie that needs a touch of sweetness, or use it to combat colds and flu.

K

Kava.* Kava root belongs to the pepper family of plants, and possesses plenty of health benefits. Kava has antimicrobial, antispasmodic, diuretic, and stimulant properties and can act as a muscle relaxant. Kava can be used for stress relief, kidney infections, fibromyalgia, and more. Avoid kava if you're pregnant or breastfeeding and don't use heavy equipment when consuming a smoothie with kava. Avoid kava if you drink alcohol or have any liver problems and do not use kava for a long period of time. You can buy dried kava root or extracts at health food stores.

L

Lavender.* Not just a great-smelling herb, lavender also has health benefits. It is a relaxant, antibacterial, and antiseptic, and can help the flow of bile in the system. It acts as a tonic to the nervous system and has been used to treat depression, indigestion, insomnia, tension, and colic. Don't use a lot of lavender if you're pregnant, since it does stimulate the uterus. Use fresh sprigs or dried lavender flowers in your smoothie for an interesting taste and lots of health benefits.

Lecithin. Lecithin can be bought in granular or capsule form. It is a source of choline, which is very beneficial to the brain. Add granules or capsules to a smoothie mixture for stronger neurons and increased memory.

Licorice.* Licorice acts as a gentle laxative, so is great for a detox smoothie. Also, licorice has anti-inflammatory, anti-arthritic, antibacterial, and expectorant properties, as well as having a calming effect on the gastric system. Licorice can also help the body expel mucus, so it is good for treating coughs and bronchitis. Avoid licorice if you have high blood pressure. To add to smoothies, simmer a chopped root in water for 8–10 minutes, then cool, strain, and throw out the root, leaving the infused liquid behind.

M

Maple Syrup. Maple syrup is a good sweetener for smoothies. It contains potassium, calcium, and thiamin. Use pure maple syrup for healthier benefits.

Marshmallow.* Marshmallow can soothe mucus membranes, which include sinuses and the digestive tract. It is a cleansing substance, so can be used to treat problems in the digestive tract, ulcers, bronchial inflammation, and more. You can use flowers, leaves, or roots, or you can make an infusion as explained for licorice, above.

Milk Thistle.* Milk thistle can protect the liver by promoting bile production and flow, and it encourages the liver to produce new cells, which has a detoxifying effect on the body. Use seeds crushed into a fine powder in your smoothie, or do an infusion if you don't want the powder.

N

Nutmeg. Nutmeg has anti-inflammatory properties, as well as digestive stimulant properties. Don't use nutmeg in large doses if you are pregnant but do use it to control stomach upset and, to some degree, muscle tension. Grind up dried nutmeg into a fine powder and add to smoothies.

O

Oats. Oats have antidepressant properties and are good for the nerves. Use the dried oat seeds or leaves by crushing them into a fine powder and adding to smoothies.

P

Parsley.* Parsley is a diuretic, so it flushes the body of extra water and purifies the kidneys. Parsley is rich in vitamin C. It is also a uterine stimulant, so avoid it in large doses if you are pregnant. Use fresh or dried parsley in your smoothie.

Peppermint. Peppermint is beneficial to the digestive tract as well as the liver. It has both antispasmodic and analgesic properties. It can soothe the stomach, stimulate the liver and gallbladder, and improve appetite. Do not give peppermint to children, and avoid it if you're pregnant. For smoothies, use fresh leaves or dried leaves.

Protein Powder. When the recipe calls for protein powder, we like soy protein powder. Because soy can increase estrogen production, it is not recommended for women who have had breast cancer or uterine cancer. In other situations, it can help lower cholesterol, help the body retain calcium, and add much-needed protein to a smoothie that is acting as a meal replacement. Choose protein powder that is made from organic, water-washed soybeans.

Psyllium.* Psyllium is good for detoxing because of its gentle laxative properties. It soothes the digestive tract even as it stimulates the intestines, so it is gentle and safe to use, though it should be avoided if you've ever exhibited an allergy to it or if you have asthma. Also, in cases of bowel obstruction, see a doctor. Don't try to use psyllium to treat a bowel obstruction. Use the seeds in smoothies, but make sure you drink plenty of water.

R

Rosemary. Rosemary has astringent, antioxidant, anti-inflammatory, and antidepressant properties, as well as being a good natural food preservative. It has been shown to fight depression and tension headaches, may help prevent breast cancer, and can help improve brain function. Don't take rosemary in large doses if you're pregnant. Use fresh sprigs in your smoothie, just pick out the stems first.

S

Sage. Sage has antibiotic, antimicrobial, antiseptic, and antioxidant properties, as well as acting as a circulatory stimulant and natural deodorant. It can cure sore throats and has also been shown to help relieve certain symptoms of menopause. Sage is a uterine stimulant, so avoid it if you're pregnant and also avoid it if you have epilepsy or high blood pressure.

Sesame Seeds. Sesame seeds are tasty, and they can act as a laxative in the system. Sesame seed oil is a good source of vitamin E and can boost the body's metabolism. Sprinkle some sesame seeds on your smoothie for a great taste and change in texture, or blend them in for a smooth smoothie.

Slippery Elm Bark. Slippery elm bark is one of the most beneficial herbs in terms of its wide-ranging health benefits. It is soothing to the digestive system, in addition to acting as a nutritive. Slippery elm bark can be used to treat ulcers, hernias, Crohn's disease, and IBS, and it can even be used as a topical paste to heal wounds. Slippery elm bark is difficult to mix into liquid, so it is great to have smoothies to blend it into for all the wonderful health benefits. Buy the dried bark in powder form and use 1 teaspoon per cup of your smoothie.

Spearmint. Spearmint is less potent than peppermint, so it is safe to use with children. Spearmint helps soothe the stomach and can help ease the woes of the common cold. Use fresh sprigs or dried flowers and leaves for your smoothie.

Spirulina. Spirulina, a highly nutritious micro saltwater plant (algae), is mostly protein, so if you can't use soy, it's a good replacement. It is a great source of essential amino acids and is thought to protect the heart during chemotherapy treatment for cancer. It may also help prevent strokes, speed up the recovery of stroke victims, and maybe even reverse memory loss. You can buy it in health food stores, and it is safe to use as long as you don't have a metabolic disorder that stops you from metabolizing phenylalanine.

Sprouts. Sprouts, as long as they are grown correctly, can add vitamins A and C and a lot of B vitamins to your smoothie. Just make sure you choose sprouts that are organic. Most people choose to grow their own sprouts to make sure they avoid the harmful bacteria found in nonorganic, mass-produced sprouts. Add a cup of sprouts to your smoothie for a green nutrition boost.

St. John's Wort. St. John's Wort has long been known for its mood-elevating properties, but it is antiviral, anti-inflammatory, and astringent. St. John's wort can reduce the effectiveness of many different drugs, so make sure you check for interactions. Use dried leaves or flowers crushed into a fine powder.

Stevia. Stevia provides natural sweetness without added calories. It also boosts energy and can help prevent cavities. It is safe sweetness as it does not raise blood sugar levels, and it may stimulate the pancreas. Stevia may be beneficial for overweight people. It is believed that a disconnect may exist between the stomach and the hypothalamus in those who are overweight, which fails to "turn off" hunger feelings when the person is full. Stevia may correct this defect and right the hunger mechanism, thus "turning off" hunger sensations when you are full.

T

Thyme. Thyme has expectorant, antiseptic, antioxidant, and antispasmodic properties. It is used mainly to treat chest infections but also can be used to treat IBS. People with thyroid problems, children, and pregnant women should avoid thyme. Use dried or fresh leaves in your smoothie.

Turmeric.* Turmeric has antimicrobial, antibacterial, antifungal, antiviral, antioxidant, anti-inflammatory, anticoagulant, and analgesic properties and is used to treat a wide variety of ailments. It is thought that turmeric fights breast and colon cancer, and it is used to treat digestive disorders. You can find turmeric in Asian grocery stores and health food stores. Add fresh or dried root to your smoothies. In a pinch you can use the dried powder version of turmeric.

V

Valerian. A soothing root, valerian has sedative properties, so it is used to treat depression, insomnia, anxiety, migraines, and high blood pressure. Not everybody reacts well to valerian, so try it out in small doses at first. Use fresh valerian root for the best results.

W

Wheat Germ. Wheat germ is a source of thiamin and vitamin E and is a smoothie staple.

Wheat Grass.* Wheat grass has antioxidant, anticancer, antibiotic, and anti-inflammatory properties and may help cleanse the blood. It's easier to use powdered wheat grass than to buy a special juicer. Start slow with wheat grass, as it can cause nausea and diarrhea in some people.

Liquids and Bases

A

Almond Milk. Great for the lactose-intolerant, almond milk is a tasty addition to smoothies that replaces milk, soy milk, or water. It is cholesterol free, and so a great alternative for people who are trying to lower their cholesterol.

C

Coconut Milk. Coconut milk comes from the meat of the coconut itself. When you grate the meat, the oil-rich liquid that comes out is the actual coconut milk. It is said that coconut milk can help balance the body's electrolytes and fight dehydration. It may also have healing properties related to the digestive tract, because of its antimicrobial properties.

H

Hemp Milk. Grinding hemp seeds that have been soaked in water makes hemp milk. The resultant liquid is nutty and full of omega-3 fatty acids, magnesium, and fiber. Theoretically, hemp is safe for people with nut allergies, unlike almond milk. As always, if you have food allergies consult your allergist before trying a new product.

O

Oat Milk. Free of lactose and milk proteins, oat milk falls in the grain milk category, which also includes rice milk. It is harder to find than rice milk.

R

Rice Milk. Rice milk looks more like "normal" milk than a lot of the milk substitutes. Rice milk has a sweet taste, but that sweetness comes from a natural process, not by artificial sweeteners. Rice milk has a higher carbohydrate count than cow's milk. Most commercial rice milks are fortified with vitamins and minerals like B vitamins, calcium, and iron.

S

Skim Milk. Skim milk is cow's milk with no fat. It does, however, still contain lactose, and is still an animal product, so not appropriate for vegans. Skim milk is high in vitamin A.

Soy Milk. Soy milk has the same amount of protein as cow's milk but is not an animal product. It has a little saturated fat and cholesterol, but nothing like whole cow's milk, and it is the go-to smoothie liquid for many people. If you have a history of breast cancer or uterine cancer, talk to your doctor before consuming soy.

T

Tofu. Tofu is made out of soybean curd and has the same health benefits and characteristics as soy and soy milk. Adding tofu to your smoothie gives it a smooth, silky texture and can add the consistency of ice cream or heavy cream, making you feel like your smoothie is naughtier than it is.

W

Water. The go-to. The essence of life. H_2O. Many of the detox smoothies you'll see here will use water only as a base. Remember, also, that on any weight loss plan or detox plan, it is vital that you consume at least 64 ounces of water per day. The rest you'll get from your smoothies, fruits, and vegetables.

Y

Yogurt. Yogurt contains lactobacilli and helps maintain bacterial balance in the intestinal tract. Yogurt helps lower blood cholesterol, has antibacterial properties, and can help build the immune system. It also adds a creamy texture to smoothies. In any recipe that calls for a dairy substitute, it is fine to use yogurt, real milk, or other dairy products if you are not vegan and do not have lactose intolerance. Conversely, soy yogurt and other nondairy yogurts are available.

weight loss smoothies

4

Get Moving Breakfast Smoothies

WHILE MAKING SMOOTHIES isn't difficult, it will help to keep some things in mind before you begin. Following these guidelines can make the difference in ending up with a beautiful smoothie with a pleasing texture or a chunky concoction that looks like something you should pour down the drain.

Adding the ingredients:

- Always pour the liquid in first. It will help prevent the blades from being stuck in the heavier, frozen bits of fruit.

- Add semisolids next such as yogurt, powders, and ice cream.

- Add fresh fruit and then any frozen fruit.

- If ice is called for, add this last always.

- If you have time, it can help to thaw fruits before adding them—you don't need fruit frozen throughout to have a good smoothie.

- Be sure to cut large pieces of fruit into smaller pieces. This will help the blades cut through easier.

- Once you decide on some of your most favorite recipes, buy in bulk. Frozen fruits work best in smoothies so don't feel you have to have fresh fruit on hand.

How to Blend

Blending a smoothie isn't rocket science but once you have added your ingredients in the correct order, using this process of blending will help keep your blender from overheating and possibly painting your walls with half-blended fruit.

Start at a lower speed. Depending on your blender the setting will vary, but slowly increasing the speed is important. Let the blades have time to grab the fruit and ice until everything is freely circulating in the blender. It can take 20–45 seconds for this to happen. Your patience will be rewarded.

After you have slowly increased the speed you should have the blender up to a full power. The ingredients should be mixed to a smooth consistency. This is when we suggest you leave it on full power for another 30–45 seconds to let air get inside your smoothie and give it a lighter consistency.

If the blender is too full, the frozen ingredients may trap the blades. If this happens, unplug the blender and use your plunger that came with your blender or a wooden spoon to dislodge the pieces. Sometimes simply adding water or more juice will also free the blades.

Merry Morning Smoothie

ADDING brewer's yeast to your morning smoothie adds chromium, which has been found to correct glucose intolerance and insulin resistance. This can decrease your appetite and help promote weight loss.

INGREDIENTS
½ cup nonfat milk
½ cup frozen strawberries
½ banana
2 tablespoons protein powder
1 tablespoon wheat germ
1 teaspoon brewer's yeast

NUTRITIONAL INFORMATION

Calories: 291	Fiber: 8 g
Carbohydrate: 37 g	Sugar: 17.9 g
Protein: 34 g	Vitamin A: 95 IU
Fat: 3.3 g	Vitamin C: 38 mg
Saturated Fat: 0.6 g	Calcium: 222 mg
Cholesterol: 2.5 mg	Iron: 7.8 mg
Sodium: 325 mg	Potassium: 684 mg

Cocoa Breakfast Smoothie

SMOOTHIES with wheat germ help add extra fiber for regularity as well as protein and vitamin E—great for assisting in weight loss.

INGREDIENTS

½ cup cocoa soy or almond milk

1 banana

1 tablespoon cocoa protein powder

1 tablespoon wheat germ

1 tablespoon brewer's yeast

½ teaspoon ground cinnamon

NUTRITIONAL INFORMATION

Calories: 229

Carbohydrate: 39 g

Protein: 13 g

Fat: 4.3 g

Saturated Fat: 0.4 g

Cholesterol: 1.8 mg

Sodium: 84 mg

Fiber: 8.2 g

Sugar: 18.4 g

Vitamin A: 306 IU

Vitamin C: 6.1 mg

Calcium: 131 mg

Iron: 6.5 mg

Potassium: 468 mg

Great Granola Goodness

YOUR GRANOLA doesn't have to come in a bowl of milk or in the shape of a bar. Mixing granola with your morning smoothie provides energy for the day, while staving off mid-morning hunger.

INGREDIENTS

1 cup nonfat milk
¼ cup low-fat granola
½ cup low-fat vanilla yogurt
1 frozen banana

NUTRITIONAL INFORMATION

Calories: 388

Carbohydrate: 68 g

Protein: 21 g

Fat: 3.8 g

Saturated Fat: 1.6 g

Cholesterol: 12.3 mg

Sodium: 214 mg

Fiber: 6.1 g

Sugar: 39 g

Vitamin A: 155 IU

Vitamin C: 17.4 mg

Calcium: 552 mg

Iron: 1.9 mg

Potassium: 1,116 mg

Jump Start Breakfast Smoothie

JUMP-START your metabolism with a protein-rich fruit and yogurt smoothie. Protein powder and yogurt supply long-term energy while the fruit gives you a burst to get going in the morning.

INGREDIENTS

1 frozen banana
½ cup frozen strawberries
6 ounces low-fat plain yogurt
1 tablespoon protein powder
1⅓ cups water
6 ice cubes

NUTRITIONAL INFORMATION

Calories: 339
Carbohydrate: 64 g
Protein: 18.4 g
Fat: 2.9 g
Saturated Fat: 1.6 g
Cholesterol: 28 mg
Sodium: 158 mg

Fiber: 7.4 g
Sugar: 44 g
Vitamin A: 125 IU
Vitamin C: 56 mg
Calcium: 369 mg
Iron: 1.4 mg
Potassium: 1,026 mg

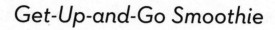

Get-Up-and-Go Smoothie

GET THE HEALTH benefits of spirulina and an energy punch with potassium, vitamins C and B$_1$, and the fatty acids in this energizing smoothie. A natural lift to start your day.

INGREDIENTS

1½ cup strawberries

1 kiwifruit

½ banana

1 tablespoon spirulina powder

1 tablespoon flax seeds

4 ice cubes

NUTRITIONAL INFORMATION

Calories: 243

Carbohydrate: 48 g

Protein: 9.1 g

Fat: 4.9 g

Saturated Fat: 0.6 g

Cholesterol: 0 mg

Sodium: 76 mg

Fiber: 10.7 g

Sugar: 27 g

Vitamin A: 105 IU

Vitamin C: 212 mg

Calcium: 115 mg

Iron: 4.1 mg

Potassium: 946 mg

Berry Good Morning Smoothie

THERE ARE few better ways to start your morning than with a berry-rich smoothie. But adding wheat germ and brewer's yeast is one way to make it even better!

INGREDIENTS

½ cup almond or soy milk

½ cup mixed frozen berries

½ banana

2 tablespoons protein powder

1 tablespoon wheat germ

1 teaspoon brewer's yeast

NUTRITIONAL INFORMATION

Calories: 347

Carbohydrate: 42 g

Protein: 34 g

Fat: 6.2 g

Saturated Fat: 1.4 g

Cholesterol: 50 mg

Sodium: 216 mg

Fiber: 10.2 g

Sugar: 18.7 g

Vitamin A: 302 IU

Vitamin C: 26 mg

Calcium: 223 mg

Iron: 7.6 mg

Potassium: 620 mg

Strawberry Morning Glory

EATING fiber and maintaining healthy weight usually go hand-in-hand. Psyllium seed powder is a wonderful source of soluble fiber to help you feel full and energized. Good news: it will help to reduce your cholesterol, too.

INGREDIENTS

1 cup frozen strawberries
6 ounces nonfat plain yogurt
½ banana
1 tablespoon brewer's yeast
1 teaspoon psyllium seed powder

NUTRITIONAL INFORMATION

Calories: 305

Carbohydrate: 60 g

Protein: 17.6 g

Fat: 1.4 g

Saturated Fat: 0.1 g

Cholesterol: 3.8 mg

Sodium: 150 mg

Fiber: 12.6 g

Sugar: 33 g

Vitamin A: 514 IU

Vitamin C: 98 mg

Calcium: 377 mg

Iron: 6.8 mg

Potassium: 574 mg

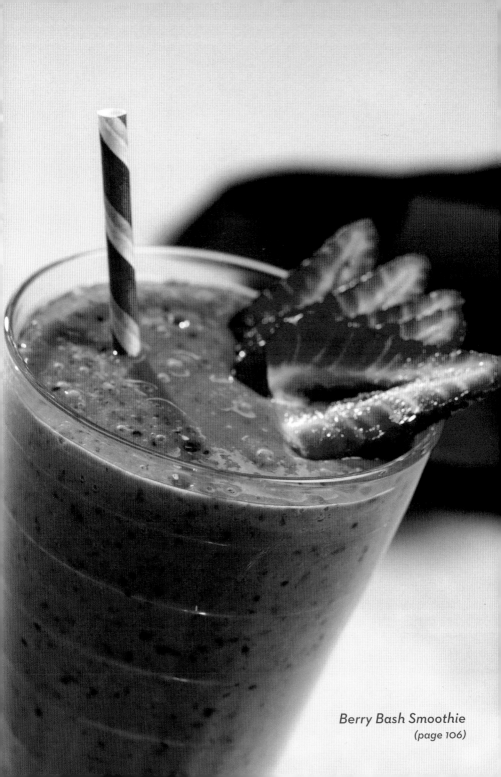

Berry Bash Smoothie
(page 106)

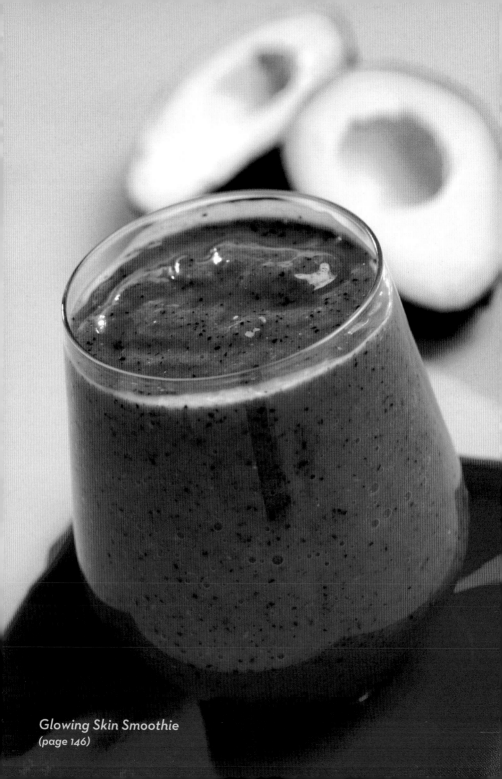

Glowing Skin Smoothie
(page 146)

Green Dew Mint Smoothie
(page 154)

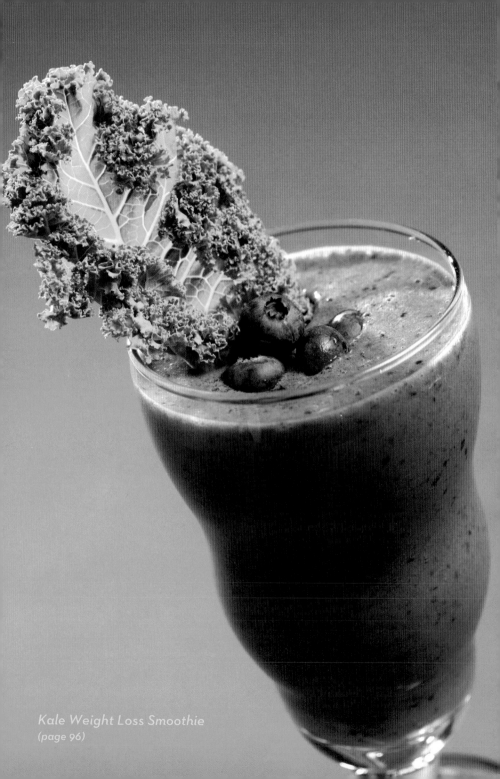

Kale Weight Loss Smoothie
(page 96)

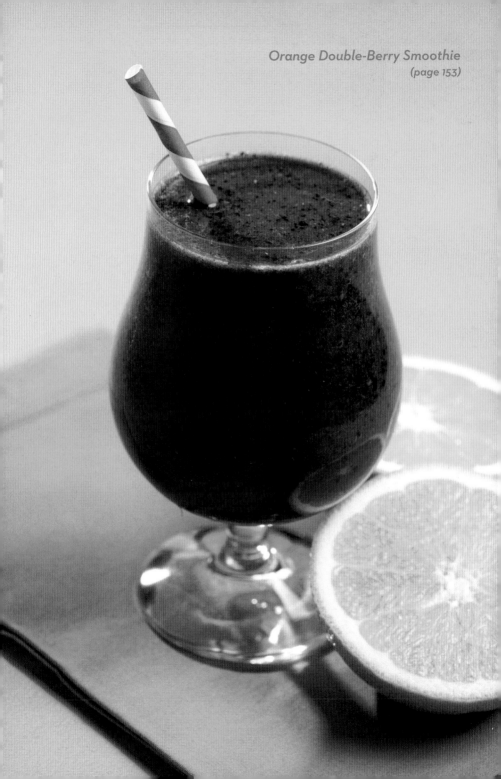

Orange Double-Berry Smoothie
(page 153)

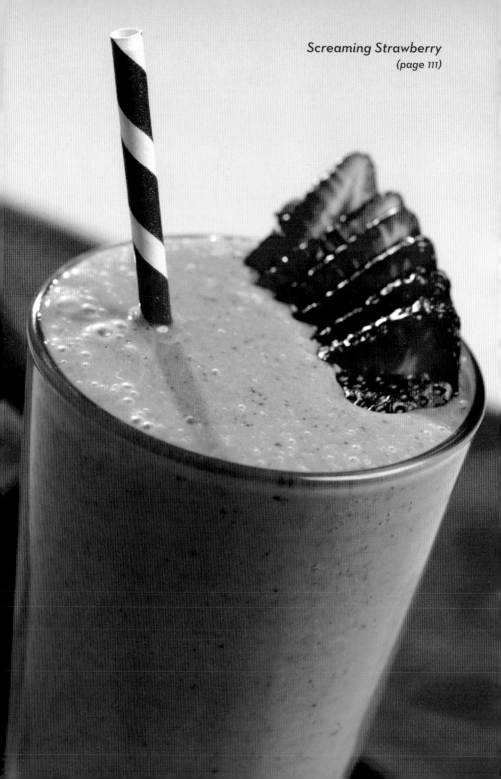

Screaming Strawberry
(page 111)

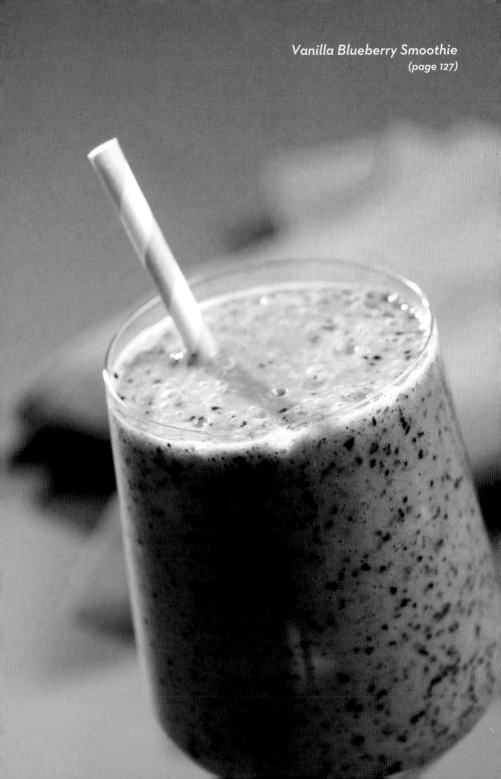

Vanilla Blueberry Smoothie
(page 127)

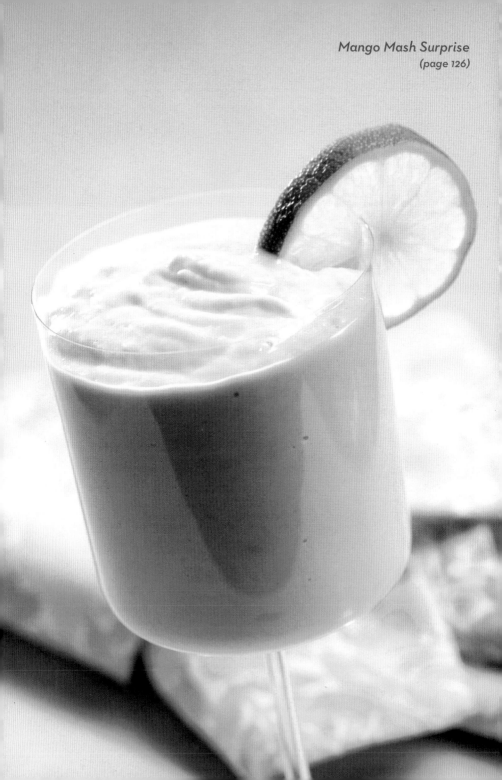

Mango Mash Surprise
(page 126)

Ruby Red Smoothie

ADDING the stevia for sweetness is optional because the kiwifruit and bananas provide their own sweet flavor which will counter the tart flavor of the grapefruit.

INGREDIENTS

1 red grapefruit (peeled and deseeded)

1 kiwifruit

1 tablespoon ground flaxseed

2 bananas

2 cups fresh baby spinach

2 teaspoons stevia (optional)

½ cup water

NUTRITIONAL INFORMATION

Calories: 392

Carbohydrate: 86 g

Protein: 9.6 g

Fat: 4.3 g

Saturated Fat: 0.6 g

Cholesterol: 0 mg

Sodium: 67 mg

Fiber: 13.4 g

Sugar: 48 g

Vitamin A: 5,901 IU

Vitamin C: 165 mg

Calcium: 179 mg

Iron: 2.7 mg

Potassium: 1,135 mg

Blueberry Almond Smoothie

SIMPLE is good sometimes. This is one of those times. Blueberries are a superfood and make any weight loss program easier and tastier. Flaxseed oil provides monounsaturated fat for added weight loss benefit.

INGREDIENTS

1 cup almond milk
1 cup frozen blueberries
1 tablespoon flaxseed oil

NUTRITIONAL INFORMATION

Calories: 250

Carbohydrate: 21 g

Protein: 2 g

Fat: 17 g

Saturated Fat: 1.5 g

Cholesterol: 0 mg

Sodium: 190 mg

Fiber: 5 g

Sugar: 13 g

Vitamin A: 500 IU

Vitamin C: 3.6 mg

Calcium: 200 mg

Iron: 0.8 mg

Potassium: 190 mg

The "Basic"
Weight Loss Smoothie

A SMOOTHIE that resembles what most people consider to be a "real" smoothie: yogurt, fruit, and optional protein powder. It's a classic combination for a good reason. It's delicious and healthy.

INGREDIENTS

½ cup skim milk

½ cup nonfat plain yogurt

1 scoop of protein powder (optional)

½ banana

1 cup fresh or frozen berries

NUTRITIONAL INFORMATION

Calories: 352

Carbohydrate: 52 g

Protein: 32 g

Fat: 2.4 g

Saturated Fat: 1.2 g

Cholesterol: 71 mg

Sodium: 191 mg

Fiber: 5.5 g

Sugar: 35 g

Vitamin A: 647 IU

Vitamin C: 18.3 mg

Calcium: 485 mg

Iron: 2 mg

Potassium: 625 mg

Sweet Molasses,
That's Good!

IF YOU LOVE bioflavonoids this smoothie is for you. Not sure what a bioflavonoid is? Well, we need them to live happy, healthy lives. They are found in citrus fruits like lemons, oranges, and grapefruits. They play an important role in the prevention and treatment of diseases such as heart disease and cancer. Don't skip the molasses, it will give this recipe a sweeter flavor and is a healthful sweetener that contains minerals that promote good health.

INGREDIENTS

½ cup orange juice

½ cup nonfat plain yogurt

½ lemon

½ grapefruit

4 ice cubes

1 ounce fresh ginger, peeled and crushed

1 tablespoon molasses

NUTRITIONAL INFORMATION

Calories: 248

Carbohydrate: 55 g

Protein: 8.5 g

Fat: 0.6 g

Saturated Fat: 0 g

Cholesterol: 2.5 mg

Sodium: 99 mg

Fiber: 3.1 g

Sugar: 39 g

Vitamin A: 1,919 IU

Vitamin C: 117 mg

Calcium: 314 mg

Iron: 1.5 mg

Potassium: 747 mg

Blackberry Ice

HIGH IN FIBER and relatively low in sugar, blackberries are a great food to help you stick to your weight-loss plan. Blackberries are about 80 percent water, making them a good fruit for those trying to lose weight. The naturally sweet flavor of the fruit helps to satisfy cravings, and the high water content helps the stomach feel full.

INGREDIENTS
1 cup frozen blackberries
1 orange
½ cup orange juice
½ grapefruit

NUTRITIONAL INFORMATION

Calories: 266	Fiber: 1.3 g
Carbohydrate: 65 g	Sugar: 47 g
Protein: 4.9 g	Vitamin A: 2,129 IU
Fat: 1.4 g	Vitamin C: 175 mg
Saturated Fat: 0 g	Calcium: 137 mg
Cholesterol: 0 mg	Iron: 1.7 mg
Sodium: 2.7 mg	Potassium: 863 mg

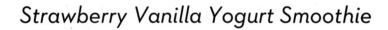

Strawberry Vanilla Yogurt Smoothie

ADDING VANILLA won't boost metabolism or help regulate blood sugars but it can help curb your cravings for chocolate and may do the same for your desire for other sweets with its aroma. Without these cravings, you are less likely to snatch the nearest sugary treat or high-calorie snack.

INGREDIENTS

1 frozen banana
6 ounces low-fat plain yogurt
1 cup frozen strawberries
1 teaspoon stevia
½ cup water
1 teaspoon vanilla
4 ice cubes

NUTRITIONAL INFORMATION

Calories: 322
Carbohydrate: 58 g
Protein: 9.1 g
Fat: 6.6 g
Saturated Fat: 3.9 g
Cholesterol: 26 mg
Sodium: 119 mg

Fiber: 7.7 g
Sugar: 35 g
Vitamin A: 400 IU
Vitamin C: 101 mg
Calcium: 267 mg
Iron: 2 mg
Potassium: 1,101 mg

Fruitful
Wheat Germ Smoothie

WHEAT GERM can provide you with fiber to give you a sense of being full and satisfying your appetite. It also contains vitamin B complex, which helps in coping with stress and benefits the metabolism. And if the body's metabolism is going strong then the body is burning more calories.

INGREDIENTS

1 ripe banana
1 cup nonfat vanilla yogurt
¼ cup orange juice
1 cup sliced peaches
¼ cup wheat germ
4 ice cubes

NUTRITIONAL INFORMATION

Calories: 414

Carbohydrate: 85 g

Protein: 18.2 g

Fat: 3.9 g

Saturated Fat: 0.6 g

Cholesterol: 6.7 mg

Sodium: 103 mg

Fiber: 10.1 g

Sugar: 51 g

Vitamin A: 1,316 IU

Vitamin C: 54 mg

Calcium: 236 mg

Iron: 3.4 mg

Potassium: 1,444 mg

5

Fill 'Er Up
Meal Replacements

Apple Pie Smoothie

THIS APPLE SMOOTHIE will have you dreaming of apple pie while giving you a delicious meal replacement containing protein-rich cashew butter. Cashew nuts are high in good fats, phytochemicals, and antioxidants and protect against cardiovascular diseases.

Apple Pie Smoothie

INGREDIENTS

½ cup skim or soy milk

6 ounces low-fat vanilla yogurt

1 teaspoon apple pie spice

1 medium apple, peeled and chopped

2 tablespoons cashew butter

4 ice cubes

NUTRITIONAL INFORMATION

Calories: 391

Carbohydrate: 53 g

Protein: 14.8 g

Fat: 16 g

Saturated Fat: 3.2 g

Cholesterol: 7.5 mg

Sodium: 144 mg

Fiber: 5.6 g

Sugar: 34 g

Vitamin A: 509 IU

Vitamin C: 13.2 mg

Calcium: 335 mg

Iron: 2.1 mg

Potassium: 608 mg

Pineapple Smoothie

THIS IS A quick and delicious smoothie that uses only four ingredients to provide a cool refreshing replacement meal. Pineapple is low in calories and energy dense. It is high in fiber and water content. Add its high level of vitamin C and you have a fruit that can aid in weight loss efforts.

INGREDIENTS

1 cup skim milk
1 cup pineapple
1 tablespoon flaxseed oil
4 ice cubes

NUTRITIONAL INFORMATION

Calories: 293

Carbohydrate: 32 g

Protein: 9.2 g

Fat: 14.6 g

Saturated Fat: 1.8 g

Cholesterol: 4.9 mg

Sodium: 129 mg

Fiber: 2.2 g

Sugar: 28 g

Vitamin A: 107 IU

Vitamin C: 77 mg

Calcium: 322 mg

Iron: 0.6 mg

Potassium: 576 mg

The Green Tart

THANKS to all its nutrients and fiber, this smoothie is very filling, so it helps keep you from having that in-between meal snack. It's a healthy meal in a smoothie with the benefit of adding spinach, providing significant dietary fiber to help you feel full for longer, which can reduce total calorie consumption.

INGREDIENTS

4 romaine lettuce leaves
2 celery stalks
1 cup fresh spinach
1 apple, peeled and chopped
1 pear
½ banana
Juice of ½ lemon
1½ cups water

NUTRITIONAL INFORMATION

Calories: 290
Carbohydrate: 75 g
Protein: 5.4 g
Fat: 1.1 g
Saturated Fat: 0.2 g
Cholesterol: 0 mg
Sodium: 128 mg

Fiber: 14.6 g
Sugar: 46 g
Vitamin A: 3,659 IU
Vitamin C: 51 mg
Calcium: 114 mg
Iron: 1.7 mg
Potassium: 1,160 mg

PB & Banana Smoothie

LOOKING for a more substantial smoothie as a meal replacement? The peanut butter smoothie will give you a healthy, fulfilling meal and a creamy nutty flavor to keep your energy levels high.

INGREDIENTS

½ cup nonfat plain yogurt

2 tablespoons creamy natural
   unsalted peanut butter

¼ very ripe banana

½ cup fat-free milk

1 tablespoon honey

4 ice cubes

NUTRITIONAL INFORMATION

Calories: 389	Fiber: 2.8 g
Carbohydrate: 45 g	Sugar: 36 g
Protein: 19.1 g	Vitamin A: 28 IU
Fat: 15.3 g	Vitamin C: 5.1 mg
Saturated Fat: 3.1 g	Calcium: 354 mg
Cholesterol: 5 mg	Iron: 4.2 mg
Sodium: 140 mg	Potassium: 575 mg

Green Mix and Mash Smoothie

THIS SMOOTHIE contains a mix of ingredients that combine a healthy dose of fruits, vegetables, herbs, and protein. You will find it hard to create a more complete meal-replacement smoothie. Parsley may aid weight-loss efforts by assisting in removing toxins from the body and aiding digestion and absorption of food nutrients.

INGREDIENTS

¼ cup grated carrot

½ cup apricots

½ papaya

1 tablespoon sesame seeds

½ avocado

1 tablespoon spirulina powder

Handful of parsley

½ cup water

NUTRITIONAL INFORMATION

Calories: 318

Carbohydrate: 31 g

Protein: 10.2 g

Fat: 21 g

Saturated Fat: 2.9 g

Cholesterol: 0 mg

Sodium: 103 mg

Fiber: 13.2 g

Sugar: 13.5 g

Vitamin A: 7,040 IU

Vitamin C: 64 mg

Calcium: 144 mg

Iron: 4.4 mg

Potassium: 1,094 mg

Strawberry Honey Smoothie

NO TIME to prepare a meal? A smoothie can be a great solution when time is lacking but a healthy meal is still desired. This smoothie makes a quick meal and gives you the protein to keep you going and feeling full without a lot of calories.

INGREDIENTS

½ cup soy milk
½ cup frozen strawberries
6 ounces low-fat vanilla yogurt
1 tablespoon honey

NUTRITIONAL INFORMATION

Calories: 305	Fiber: 3 g
Carbohydrate: 58 g	Sugar: 45 g
Protein: 12.5 g	Vitamin A: 53 IU
Fat: 4.2 g	Vitamin C: 47 mg
Saturated Fat: 1.3 g	Calcium: 298 mg
Cholesterol: 10 mg	Iron: 2 mg
Sodium: 155 mg	Potassium: 308 mg

Fruity Ice Storm

THIS PERFECT storm of flavors is also a perfect meal replacement at around 300 calories. This is guaranteed to satisfy your sweet tooth without the high calories. Molasses is a good source of copper and manganese, and the calcium in molasses may also help you lose weight.

INGREDIENTS

¼ cup unsweetened orange juice

1 banana

3 pineapple rings

½ cup unsweetened apple juice

8 ice cubes

1 teaspoon molasses (optional)

NUTRITIONAL INFORMATION

Calories: 306

Carbohydrate: 77 g

Protein: 1.4 g

Fat: 0.5 g

Saturated Fat: 0.1 g

Cholesterol: 0 mg

Sodium: 13.8 mg

Fiber: 4.7 g

Sugar: 61 g

Vitamin A: 76 IU

Vitamin C: 82 mg

Calcium: 92 mg

Iron: 2.1 mg

Potassium: 1,026 mg

Your receipt
Summer is here, and so is our Summer Reading Adventure. A fun, curious and entertaining adventure awaits you and your family. Registration begins May 14 at your library or online at www.MyLibrary.us.

Items that you checked out

Title:
Lean for life : the cookbook : the Louise Parker method.
Due: Tuesday, July 31, 2018

Title:
Skinny smoothies : 101 delicious drinks that help you detox and lose weight / Shell Harris and Eliza
Due: Tuesday, July 31, 2018

Title: My paleo patisserie / Jenni Hulet ; foreword by Danielle Walker.
Due: Tuesday, July 31, 2018

Total items: 3
Account balance: $0.00
7/10/2018 2:55 PM
Ready for pickup: 0

Questions? Call 1-888-861-READ(7323) or visit us at www.MyLibrary.us

Peach Almond Swirl

THE FLAVOR of almond adds a surprise to this peach smoothie. Rich in fiber, it will fill you up and keep your energy level high. Ounce-for-ounce, almonds are the most nutrient-dense nut.

INGREDIENTS

1 cup almond milk

½ cup frozen peaches

1 teaspoon spirulina powder

1 teaspoon psyllium seed powder

1 drop pure almond extract

NUTRITIONAL INFORMATION

Calories: 89

Carbohydrate: 14.1 g

Protein: 2.3 g

Fat: 3.2 g

Saturated Fat: 0.1 g

Cholesterol: 0 mg

Sodium: 209 mg

Fiber: 6.6 g

Sugar: 4.6 g

Vitamin A: 763 IU

Vitamin C: 84 mg

Calcium: 213 mg

Iron: 2 mg

Potassium: 411 mg

Kale Weight Loss Smoothie

FOR A GREEN, kale is unusually high in fiber, which helps you feel full. Kale is an excellent source of nutrients, especially vitamin A and calcium. With a potent combination of vitamins, minerals, and phytonutrients, kale is a dieter's friend.

INGREDIENTS

½ cup kale (leaves only)
½ cup frozen mixed berries
½ banana
½ cup rice or soy milk
¼ cup apple juice
Cinnamon, to taste

NUTRITIONAL INFORMATION

Calories: 191

Carbohydrate: 44 g

Protein: 2.4 g

Fat: 1.8 g

Saturated Fat: 0.2 g

Cholesterol: 0 mg

Sodium: 61 mg

Fiber: 4.3 g

Sugar: 18.6 g

Vitamin A: 5,192 IU

Vitamin C: 47 mg

Calcium: 62 mg

Iron: 1.1 mg

Potassium: 574 mg

Pineapple Colada

THE HEALTH benefits of coconut milk are impressive and for an added bonus, it may increase thermogenesis, the process in which your body metabolizes fats. Either way you'll love the taste!

INGREDIENTS
1½ cups chopped pineapple
1 cup low-fat milk
¼ cup light coconut milk
10 ice cubes

NUTRITIONAL INFORMATION

Calories: 283	Fiber: 3.3 g
Carbohydrate: 43 g	Sugar: 36 g
Protein: 9.4 g	Vitamin A: 596 IU
Fat: 9.1 g	Vitamin C: 112 mg
Saturated Fat: 6.1 g	Calcium: 316 mg
Cholesterol: 19.5 mg	Iron: 0.8 mg
Sodium: 114 mg	Potassium: 619 mg

Peachy Keen Smoothie

SHORT ON TIME, but still want great flavor? Try this one-fruit smoothie—it will give you the sweet taste of peach and the nutty flavor of almonds in one delicious drink. Essential oils in flax seeds help the stomach to hold food longer and slow digestion, which helps regulate insulin levels.

INGREDIENTS
1 cup almond milk
1 banana
1 cup frozen unsweetened peaches
2 teaspoons flaxseed oil

NUTRITIONAL INFORMATION

Calories: 455	Fiber: 6.1 g
Carbohydrate: 42 g	Sugar: 23 g
Protein: 3.3 g	Vitamin A: 976 IU
Fat: 31 g	Vitamin C: 88 mg
Saturated Fat: 3.1 g	Calcium: 206 mg
Cholesterol: 0 mg	Iron: 0.7 mg
Sodium: 181 mg	Potassium: 612 mg

Power Strawberry Smoothie

DON'T UNDERESTIMATE this two-fruit smoothie. The fruits get a big healthy boost from the flaxseed oil and brewer's yeast, which will help you keep a healthy weight. Research shows that protein is more filling than fat or carbs, which makes it an important factor in regulating your appetite and avoiding hunger cravings.

INGREDIENTS

1½ cups frozen strawberries
1 cup orange juice
1 tablespoon protein powder
1 tablespoon flaxseed oil
1 tablespoon brewer's yeast

NUTRITIONAL INFORMATION

Calories: 470	Fiber: 11 g
Carbohydrate: 63 g	Sugar: 36 g
Protein: 21 g	Vitamin A: 645 IU
Fat: 16.6 g	Vitamin C: 261 mg
Saturated Fat: 2.1 g	Calcium: 151 mg
Cholesterol: 16.6 mg	Iron: 7.5 mg
Sodium: 40 mg	Potassium: 1,075 mg

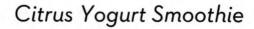

Citrus Yogurt Smoothie

CITRUS FRUITS combine for a zesty and tangy flavor in this smoothie that is also high in vitamin C. The monounsaturated fat in soy milk prevents increase of blood fat and inhibits your intestinal fat and cholesterol absorption.

INGREDIENTS

1 cup soy milk
6 ounces low-fat lemon yogurt
1 medium orange peeled, cleaned,
and sliced into sections
1 tablespoon flaxseed oil
4 ice cubes

NUTRITIONAL INFORMATION

Calories: 489

Carbohydrate: 61 g

Protein: 15.2 g

Fat: 21 g

Saturated Fat: 3.1 g

Cholesterol: 11.2 mg

Sodium: 215 mg

Fiber: 4.6 g

Sugar: 48 g

Vitamin A: 377 IU

Vitamin C: 72 mg

Calcium: 301 mg

Iron: 1.7 mg

Potassium: 526 mg

Apple Raspberry Smoothie

GRAPES can hinder any weight loss plan, as they only provide simple carbohydrates and are sugary. The key, as with most things in life, is moderation. Half a cup of red grapes will give this smoothie a touch of sweetness and provide more than a handful of healthy heart benefits without sabotaging your weight loss efforts.

INGREDIENTS

1 banana

2 apples

½ cup red grapes

½ cup raspberries

½ cup water

4 ice cubes

NUTRITIONAL INFORMATION

Calories: 382

Carbohydrate: 99 g

Protein: 3.6 g

Fat: 1.5 g

Saturated Fat: 0.2 g

Cholesterol: 0 mg

Sodium: 7 mg

Fiber: 16.5 g

Sugar: 67 g

Vitamin A: 345 IU

Vitamin C: 52 mg

Calcium: 51 mg

Iron: 1.4 mg

Potassium: 1,058 mg

Chocolate, Peanut Butter, and Banana Smoothie

THIS SMOOTHIE will satisfy you on those days when you want the rich taste of chocolate. And what goes better with chocolate than peanut butter? The high protein in this smoothie makes it a great breakfast choice that will fulfill your appetite until lunch. With less than 250 calories, this is a rich-tasting smoothie that is surprisingly low in calories.

INGREDIENTS

½ banana
1 tablespoon natural peanut butter
½ cup nonfat milk
2 tablespoons chocolate whey protein
6 ice cubes

NUTRITIONAL INFORMATION

Calories: 325
Carbohydrate: 27 g
Protein: 30 g
Fat: 10.9 g
Saturated Fat: 3.2 g
Cholesterol: 43 mg
Sodium: 157 mg

Fiber: 6.5 g
Sugar: 16.4 g
Vitamin A: 46 IU
Vitamin C: 6.3 mg
Calcium: 304 mg
Iron: 1.4 mg
Potassium: 660 mg

Mocha Cocoa Madness

EVERY SMOOTHIE book should have at least one coffee smoothie, and here is ours. The cocoa powder adds a chocolate flavor that makes this smoothie seem far more decadent than it is. Even better, researchers reported the ability of cocoa to interfere with the ability of the body to metabolize dietary fat into fatty tissue.

INGREDIENTS
6 ounces low-fat vanilla yogurt
1 shot espresso (decaffeinated or regular)
2 teaspoons cocoa powder
4 ice cubes

NUTRITIONAL INFORMATION

Calories: 162	Fiber: 1.8 g
Carbohydrate: 27 g	Sugar: 24 g
Protein: 9.5 g	Vitamin A: 73 IU
Fat: 2.8 g	Vitamin C: 1.4 mg
Saturated Fat: 1.8 g	Calcium: 298 mg
Cholesterol: 8.5 mg	Iron: 0.9 mg
Sodium: 113 mg	Potassium: 455 mg

6

Get Moving
Energy Smoothies

Berry Bash Smoothie

THIS BERRY-RICH smoothie is an excellent source of potassium. Potassium helps to build muscles, helps muscle work properly, and helps convert the food we eat into energy. It is particularly important when trying to achieve weight loss goals.

Berry Bash Smoothie

INGREDIENTS

1 cup almond or soy milk
½ cup frozen mixed berries
½ banana
2 tablespoons protein powder
1 teaspoon brewer's yeast

NUTRITIONAL INFORMATION

Calories: 315
Carbohydrate: 38 g
Protein: 28 g
Fat: 5.8 g
Saturated Fat: 1 g
Cholesterol: 46 mg
Sodium: 266 mg

Fiber: 8 g
Sugar: 22 g
Vitamin A: 538 IU
Vitamin C: 5.1 mg
Calcium: 294 mg
Iron: 5.8 mg
Potassium: 480 mg

Apricot Energy Punch

THE HOT FLAVOR of ginger complements the sweeter taste of apricots. Spinach, celery, and apple give this smoothie plenty of vitamins and minerals great for weight loss and increased energy.

INGREDIENTS

4 apricots
1 apple
1 small stalk celery
2 cups fresh baby spinach
1 tablespoon peeled, grated ginger root
4 ice cubes

NUTRITIONAL INFORMATION

Calories: 208
Carbohydrate: 47 g
Protein: 6.1 g
Fat: 1.2 g
Saturated Fat: 0.2 g
Cholesterol: 0 mg
Sodium: 84 mg

Fiber: 9.2 g
Sugar: 32 g
Vitamin A: 6,879 IU
Vitamin C: 35 mg
Calcium: 102 mg
Iron: 2.5 mg
Potassium: 674 mg

Banana Tofu Smoothie

TOFU WILL add a creamy texture and a good amount of protein to help you feel full and give you sustained energy. Tofu absorbs flavors, so adding cinnamon gives this smoothie flavor with more spice, with the added benefit that cinnamon can alter your metabolism from fat-making to fat-burning mode by increasing insulin sensitivity.

INGREDIENTS
½ cup low-fat milk
¼ cup silken tofu, drained
½ ripe banana
1 tablespoon sugar
1 teaspoon instant coffee powder,
    preferably espresso
2 ice cubes
½ teaspoon cinnamon

NUTRITIONAL INFORMATION

Calories: 165

Carbohydrate: 26 g

Protein: 7.5 g

Fat: 4.1 g

Saturated Fat: 1.8 g

Cholesterol: 9.8 mg

Sodium: 54 mg

Fiber: 1.6 g

Sugar: 18.3 g

Vitamin A: 268 IU

Vitamin C: 5.3 mg

Calcium: 165 mg

Iron: 0.8 mg

Potassium: 549 mg

Orange Dream Smoothie

THE SWEET POTATOES do double duty by making the smoothie extra sweet and extra creamy! Thanks to their carotenoids, sweet potatoes stabilize blood sugar and lower insulin resistance, supplying energy *and* helping weight loss!

INGREDIENTS

1 frozen banana
1 orange
1 cup soy milk
¼ cup cooked, mashed sweet potatoes
½ cup nonfat vanilla yogurt

NUTRITIONAL INFORMATION

Calories: 426

Carbohydrate: 86 g

Protein: 13.8 g

Fat: 4.9 g

Saturated Fat: 0.6 g

Cholesterol: 3.3 mg

Sodium: 198 mg

Fiber: 8.7 mg

Sugar: 57 g

Vitamin A: 6,382 IU

Vitamin C: 82 mg

Calcium: 253 mg

Iron: 2 mg

Potassium: 949 mg

Peachy Fling

A HIGH-ENERGY smoothie that will get you moving, or better yet, keep you moving. Brewer's yeast adds an important weight management component to this smoothie. Brewer's yeast is a nutritional supplement derived from a single-celled fungus containing high amounts of chromium, protein, and B vitamins. This makes brewer's yeast a useful tool in weight loss.

INGREDIENTS

1 cup peaches

6 ounces nonfat lemon yogurt

1 to 2 tablespoons protein powder

1 teaspoon brewer's yeast

NUTRITIONAL INFORMATION

Calories: 268

Carbohydrate: 31 g

Protein: 30 g

Fat: 2.7 g

Saturated Fat: 1 g

Cholesterol: 55 mg

Sodium: 202 mg

Fiber: 3.3 g

Sugar: 22 g

Vitamin A: 1,070 IU

Vitamin C: 6.5 mg

Calcium: 256 mg

Iron: 3.2 mg

Potassium: 593 mg

Screaming Strawberry

THIS SMOOTHIE is a classic recipe with the bonus energy from the protein powder and brewer's yeast. Go get 'em!

INGREDIENTS

1 cup frozen strawberries

6 ounces nonfat strawberry yogurt

1 teaspoon brewer's yeast

1 teaspoon soy protein powder

1 teaspoon flaxseed oil

4 ice cubes

NUTRITIONAL INFORMATION

Calories: 257

Carbohydrate: 39 g

Protein: 10.7 g

Fat: 7.7 g

Saturated Fat: 0.8 g

Cholesterol: 5 mg

Sodium: 101 mg

Fiber: 6.4 g

Sugar: 21 g

Vitamin A: 500 IU

Vitamin C: 92 mg

Calcium: 185 mg

Iron: 4.2 mg

Potassium: 570 mg

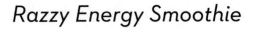

Razzy Energy Smoothie

THIS SMOOTHIE is great after a workout. Raspberries are high in salicylates, which are known for reducing aches and pains. The banana will replace your lost potassium, and glucose from the orange will help reenergize muscles.

INGREDIENTS

1 cup frozen raspberries
1 cup almond milk
½ frozen banana
2 tablespoons orange juice concentrate

NUTRITIONAL INFORMATION

Calories: 175

Carbohydrate: 35 g

Protein: 3.7 g

Fat: 3.2 g

Saturated Fat: 0.1 g

Cholesterol: 0 mg

Sodium: 185 mg

Fiber: 7.5 g

Sugar: 17.1 g

Vitamin A: 738 IU

Vitamin C: 30 mg

Calcium: 243 mg

Iron: 2 mg

Potassium: 401 mg

Frothing Berry Smoothie

POTASSIUM helps with muscle development, metabolism, energy production, blood pressure regulation, and other vital components for keeping a healthy weight. This smoothie is loaded with potassium, giving your muscles and your diet extra *oomph*.

INGREDIENTS

1 cup light soy milk
½ cup frozen mixed berries
½ frozen banana
2 tablespoons protein powder
1 teaspoon lecithin granules
1 teaspoon brewer's yeast

NUTRITIONAL INFORMATION

Calories: 355
Carbohydrate: 39 g
Protein: 32 g
Fat: 6.9 g
Saturated Fat: 1.6 g
Cholesterol: 50 mg
Sodium: 243 mg

Fiber: 6.9 g
Sugar: 24 g
Vitamin A: 538 IU
Vitamin C: 25 mg
Calcium: 416 mg
Iron: 5 mg
Potassium: 688 mg

Greek Greenie

KEEP YOUR BODY energized with this smoothie. It provides defense against muscle fatigue with nutrients like malic acid, calcium, magnesium, and creatine, which is a nitrogenous organic acid that occurs naturally in the human body. Creatine increases the body's ability to produce energy rapidly. With more energy, you can train harder and more often, producing faster results.

INGREDIENTS
1 cup unsweetened apple juice
½ cup nonfat plain Greek yogurt
4 ice cubes
2 tablespoons lemon juice
¼ teaspoon creatine powder
1 teaspoon liquid chlorophyll

NUTRITIONAL INFORMATION

Calories: 210	Fiber: 0.3 g
Carbohydrate: 41 g	Sugar: 38 g
Protein: 6.2 g	Vitamin A: 254 IU
Fat: 0.3 g	Vitamin C: 6.1 mg
Saturated Fat: 0.1 g	Calcium: 243 mg
Cholesterol: 2.5 mg	Iron: 0.9 mg
Sodium: 133 mg	Potassium: 302 mg

Cherry Buzz

CHERRIES HAVE high levels of disease-fighting antioxidants and contain important nutrients such as beta-carotene, vitamin C, potassium, iron, magnesium, and folate. Besides being great for you, they have a wonderful tart flavor that will keep your lips smacking.

INGREDIENTS

1 cup frozen cherries
½ cup orange juice
½ lemon
¼ cup water
1 tablespoon honey

NUTRITIONAL INFORMATION

Calories: 218
Carbohydrate: 55 g
Protein: 3.3 g
Fat: 0.4 g
Saturated Fat: 0 g
Cholesterol: 0 mg
Sodium: 2.6 mg

Fiber: 4.1 g
Sugar: 46 g
Vitamin A: 554 IU
Vitamin C: 79 mg
Calcium: 22 mg
Iron: 1 mg
Potassium: 299 mg

Red Cabbage Satisfaction

CABBAGE is a low-calorie, high-fiber food, and those two characteristics make it a dieter's friend. An added bonus is the fact that red cabbage is rich in natural pigments called anthocyanins, which new research suggests may help boost insulin production and lower blood-sugar levels. Cabbage is so low in calories that some call it a negative-calorie food, because it may burn more calories to digest than it provides your body.

INGREDIENTS

3 cups of red cabbage
1 frozen banana
1 cup frozen strawberries
½ cup frozen raspberries
1 teaspoon stevia
2 ice cubes
1 cup water

NUTRITIONAL INFORMATION

Calories: 360

Carbohydrate: 75 g

Protein: 7.1 g

Fat: 1 g

Saturated Fat: 0.2 g

Cholesterol: 0 mg

Sodium: 78 mg

Fiber: 15.8 g

Sugar: 38 g

Vitamin A: 3,255 IU

Vitamin C: 264 mg

Calcium: 182 mg

Iron: 48 mg

Potassium: 1,398 mg

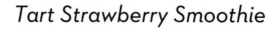

Tart Strawberry Smoothie

THE ACIDIC flavor of lemon juice contrasts wonderfully with the sweet taste of strawberries, making this recipe one of our favorites and it has less than 250 calories.

INGREDIENTS

1 large ripe banana

1½ cups frozen strawberries

1 teaspoon stevia

1 teaspoon lemon juice

1 cup water

4 ice cubes

NUTRITIONAL INFORMATION

Calories: 239

Carbohydrate: 62 g

Protein: 2.9 g

Fat: 0.9 g

Saturated Fat: 0.2 g

Cholesterol: 0 mg

Sodium: 8.1 mg

Fiber: 10.5 g

Sugar: 32 g

Vitamin A: 237 IU

Vitamin C: 151 mg

Calcium: 60 mg

Iron: 2.9 mg

Potassium: 985 mg

Honey of a Smoothie

MELONS provide a healthy dose of fiber and their sweet flavor is a good substitute for high-calorie snacks. Kiwifruit is an excellent source of dietary fiber good for filling you up and suppressing your appetite.

INGREDIENTS

2 cups honeydew melon
2 kiwifruits
1 green apple, peeled
1 tablespoon lime juice
1 teaspoon stevia
4 ice cubes

NUTRITIONAL INFORMATION

Calories: 301

Carbohydrate: 77 g

Protein: 3.6 g

Fat: 1.3 g

Saturated Fat: 0.1 g

Cholesterol: 0 mg

Sodium: 68 mg

Fiber: 12.4 g

Sugar: 60 g

Vitamin A: 412 IU

Vitamin C: 218 mg

Calcium: 94 mg

Iron: 1.5 mg

Potassium: 1,287 mg

Alpha Beta Smoothie

ONE OF CARROTS' fat-fighting features is their high fiber content, not to mention loads of beta-carotene, which aids the body by helping fight many illnesses and diseases such as diabetes, arthritis, and cancers.

INGREDIENTS

2 apricots
½ frozen papaya
½ frozen mango
1 small carrot
1 tablespoon honey

NUTRITIONAL INFORMATION

Calories: 247

Carbohydrate: 62 g

Protein: 1.4 g

Fat: 1 g

Saturated Fat: 0.01 g

Cholesterol: 0 mg

Sodium: 39 mg

Fiber: 7.1 g

Sugar: 51 g

Vitamin A: 12,266 IU

Vitamin C: 132 mg

Calcium: 66 mg

Iron: 0.6 mg

Potassium: 716 mg

7

Kick Midafternoon Slump Smoothies

Blue Peach Smoothie

BLUE SMOOTHIES are beautiful and tasty. A generous dose of protein from the wheat germ and almond milk will make your morning energy spike or give you a boost in the middle of the afternoon. Low calories and high energy are a great combo for this smoothie.

Blue Peach Smoothie

INGREDIENTS

1 cup frozen blueberries
1 peach
6 ounces nonfat peach yogurt
⅓ cup almond milk
1 tablespoon wheat germ

NUTRITIONAL INFORMATION

Calories: 275

Carbohydrate: 52 g

Protein: 12 g

Fat: 3.7 g

Saturated Fat: 0.4 g

Cholesterol: 5 mg

Sodium: 147 mg

Fiber: 8.1 g

Sugar: 34 g

Vitamin A: 672 IU

Vitamin C: 13.7 mg

Calcium: 292 mg

Iron: 1.9 mg

Potassium: 468 mg

Tropical Ginger Smoothie

THIS SMOOTHIE contains medium-chain fatty acids (MCFAs) from the coconut milk, a unique fat that is sent straight to the liver and immediately burned for fuel. Research shows this quick path can speed the metabolic rate by up to 50 percent.

INGREDIENTS

½ cup apple juice

1 tablespoon coconut milk

1 banana

½ cup pineapple chunks

¼ teaspoon grated, peeled ginger root

4 ice cubes

NUTRITIONAL INFORMATION

Calories: 268

Carbohydrate: 59 g

Protein: 1.7 g

Fat: 4.1 g

Saturated Fat: 3.3 g

Cholesterol: 0 mg

Sodium: 7.3 mg

Fiber: 4.5 g

Sugar: 44 g

Vitamin A: 77 IU

Vitamin C: 54 mg

Calcium: 17.1 mg

Iron: 1.5 mg

Potassium: 762 mg

Cantaloupe Swirl

MELONS give you the taste satisfaction of eating a dessert without the calories that usually come along with such treats. The water and fiber in this cantaloupe will add bulk to your diet, filling you up with fewer calories. Fiber in this fruit as well as in all fruits and vegetables extends digestion, keeping you feeling full for lengthier periods of time.

INGREDIENTS

1 banana

¼ ripe cantaloupe, seeded and coarsely chopped

½ cup nonfat plain yogurt

2 tablespoons nonfat dry milk

1½ tablespoons frozen orange juice concentrate

2 teaspoons honey

½ teaspoon vanilla extract

NUTRITIONAL INFORMATION

Calories: 333

Carbohydrate: 81 g

Protein: 7.9 g

Fat: 0.6 g

Saturated Fat: 0.2 g

Cholesterol: 2.5 mg

Sodium: 98 mg

Fiber: 4.1 g

Sugar: 65 g

Vitamin A: 3,806 IU

Vitamin C: 55 mg

Calcium: 216 mg

Iron: 0.5 mg

Potassium: 975 mg

Melon Tart Smoothie

THE SWEET taste of the honeydew melon marries very well with the citrus flavor of lime. This smoothie has nutrients that provide for a recovery from exercise or a good start for your busy day.

INGREDIENTS
½ cup chopped honeydew melon
1 kiwifruit
½ ripe banana, sliced
¼ cup white grape juice
1 teaspoon lime juice
2 tablespoons lemon sorbet
¼ cup ice

NUTRITIONAL INFORMATION

Calories: 200	Fiber: 4.2 g
Carbohydrate: 50 g	Sugar: 31 g
Protein: 2.1 g	Vitamin A: 84 IU
Fat: 0.8 g	Vitamin C: 113 mg
Saturated Fat: 0.1 g	Calcium: 54 mg
Cholesterol: 0 mg	Iron: 0.9 mg
Sodium: 19.9 mg	Potassium: 752 mg

Mango Mash Surprise

THE SURPRISE is the delightful creaminess the avocado brings to this smoothie and the fact that the avocado is high in monounsaturated fat. Research indicates monounsaturated fats are beneficial for weight control because they have beneficial effects on how your body uses blood sugar.

INGREDIENTS

½ cup mango
¼ cup mashed ripe avocado
6 ounces nonfat vanilla yogurt
1 tablespoon freshly squeezed lime juice
4–6 ice cubes

NUTRITIONAL INFORMATION

Calories: 215	Fiber: 4 g
Carbohydrate: 37 g	Sugar: 27 g
Protein: 6.2 g	Vitamin A: 1,438 IU
Fat: 5.7 g	Vitamin C: 28 mg
Saturated Fat: 0.9 g	Calcium: 214 mg
Cholesterol: 5 mg	Iron: 0.3 mg
Sodium: 89 mg	Potassium: 317 mg

Vanilla Blueberry Smoothie

FEATURING the smooth taste of vanilla blended with the sweet flavor of blueberries, this nutrient-rich smoothie is sure to be a favorite. Studies have shown that blueberries can reduce belly fat, improve blood sugar, and lower cholesterol levels.

INGREDIENTS

1 cup soy milk
6 ounces low-fat vanilla yogurt
1 cup frozen blueberries
1 tablespoon flaxseed oil

NUTRITIONAL INFORMATION

Calories: 422

Carbohydrate: 47 g

Protein: 15 g

Fat: 18.3 g

Saturated Fat: 2 g

Cholesterol: 5 mg

Sodium: 225 mg

Fiber: 5.5 g

Sugar: 31 g

Vitamin A: 508 IU

Vitamin C: 3.6 mg

Calcium: 211 mg

Iron: 2 mg

Potassium: 539 mg

Green Berry Smoothie

A SLY MIXTURE of greens and berries makes this a unique smoothie with more nutrients than most and with a great taste, too. This is a powerful smoothie that will make your day a little greener. Kale is high in fiber, and this fiber helps fill you up and regulate digestion, preventing the bloating and water retention that can add weight.

INGREDIENTS

½ cup frozen raspberries
½ cup frozen blueberries
1 cup apple juice
Handful of fresh spinach
2–3 leaves kale
Handful of parsley
Slice of fresh ginger
¼ tablespoon spirulina powder

NUTRITIONAL INFORMATION

Calories: 258	Fiber: 8 g
Carbohydrate: 59 g	Sugar: 39 g
Protein: 6.7 g	Vitamin A: 12,804 IU
Fat: 1.6 g	Vitamin C: 258 mg
Saturated Fat: 0.2 g	Calcium: 240 mg
Cholesterol: 0 mg	Iron: 5.4 mg
Sodium: 102 mg	Potassium: 1,043 mg

Pears, Pineapples, and Greens, Oh My!

BROCCOLI in a smoothie? Yes, and you probably won't even taste it, but you will reap the benefits of its nutrients. Broccoli is high in the vitamin C that bodies need to effectively absorb the calcium we eat, and studies indicate that calcium aids in weight loss.

INGREDIENTS

1 pear, sliced
½ cup mango
1 cup pineapple
½ cup raw broccoli
½ kiwifruit
Handful of parsley

NUTRITIONAL INFORMATION

Calories: 289
Carbohydrate: 73 g
Protein: 5.3 g
Fat: 1.6 g
Saturated Fat: 0.2 g
Cholesterol: 0 mg
Sodium: 53 mg

Fiber: 13 g
Sugar: 49 g
Vitamin A: 6,088 IU
Vitamin C: 259 mg
Calcium: 167 mg
Iron: 5.1 mg
Potassium: 1,087 mg

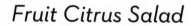

Fruit Citrus Salad

STRAWBERRIES add a sweet note to this tart fruit salad smoothie. Research indicates a physiological link between grapefruit and insulin, as the latter relates to weight management. Researchers speculate that the chemical properties of grapefruit reduce insulin levels and encourage weight loss. Good news for the grapefruit.

INGREDIENTS

1 cup strawberries
½ cup ice
1 navel orange
½ lemon
¼ grapefruit

NUTRITIONAL INFORMATION

Calories: 151

Carbohydrate: 39 g

Protein: 3.1 g

Fat: 0.9 g

Saturated Fat: 0 g

Cholesterol: 0 mg

Sodium: 3.5 mg

Fiber: 7.9 g

Sugar: 24 g

Vitamin A: 1,078 IU

Vitamin C: 207 mg

Calcium: 106 mg

Iron: 1.1 mg

Potassium: 588 mg

Creamy Mint Tea

MINT ISN'T A flavor found in smoothies that often, but you'll find it refreshing and wonder how you lived so long without it. Ginseng helps control your levels of insulin, helping you break down blood sugars at a normal pace, which helps control the way you eat.

INGREDIENTS
1½ cups brewed green tea (cool first)
6 ounces low-fat plain yogurt
4 mint leaves
2 figs
Liquid ginseng supplement
   (see label for dosage)

NUTRITIONAL INFORMATION

Calories: 236

Carbohydrate: 46 g

Protein: 9.6 g

Fat: 2.3 g

Saturated Fat: 1.1 g

Cholesterol: 10 mg

Sodium: 91 mg

Fiber: 2.9 g

Sugar: 37 g

Vitamin A: 142 IU

Vitamin C: 3.8 mg

Calcium: 285 mg

Iron: 0.8 mg

Potassium: 232 mg

Orange Melon Slush

MELONS provide fiber (good for you) with flavor (good to have) with low calories (good to hear).

INGREDIENTS

1 cup frozen honeydew or cantaloupe chunks

½ cup orange juice

½ cup mineral or filtered water

NUTRITIONAL INFORMATION

Calories: 120

Carbohydrate: 29 g

Protein: 1.9 g

Fat: 0.6 g

Saturated Fat: 0.1 g

Cholesterol: 0 mg

Sodium: 33 mg

Fiber: 1.7 g

Sugar: 25 g

Vitamin A: 337 IU

Vitamin C: 94 mg

Calcium: 24 mg

Iron: 0.6 mg

Potassium: 652 mg

Popeye's Dream Smoothie

NOT EVERYONE is as big a fan of spinach as Popeye, but you can certainly get the benefits of this leafy green without the taste that some people dislike. Spinach contains lipoic acid, which may help regulate blood-sugar levels. Including spinach in a weight-loss plan will ensure that you get a dose of nutrients including antioxidants; vitamins A, C, E, and K; coenzyme Q-10; B vitamins; and minerals like calcium, magnesium, iron, and zinc.

INGREDIENTS

1 large ripe banana
1 cup frozen blueberries
½ cup frozen strawberries
4 ounces (2 cups) fresh spinach
1 cup water

NUTRITIONAL INFORMATION

Calories: 265
Carbohydrate: 64 g
Protein: 5.9 g
Fat: 2 g
Saturated Fat: 0.4 g
Cholesterol: 0 mg
Sodium: 95 mg

Fiber: 12.5 g
Sugar: 35 g
Vitamin A: 10,842 IU
Vitamin C: 93 mg
Calcium: 149 mg
Iron: 4.6 mg
Potassium: 1,367 mg

"Lettuce" Enjoy This Smoothie

GET YOUR SALAD in a glass with this refreshing and tasty smoothie. With less than 200 calories and full of wonderful flavors and textures, you will be surprised how filling this smoothie can be.

INGREDIENTS

**1 small head of romaine lettuce,
cut in small chunks
¾ cup frozen blueberries
½ cup frozen mango
½ cup frozen cherries
1 cup water**

NUTRITIONAL INFORMATION

Calories: 188

Carbohydrate: 45 g

Protein: 3.8 g

Fat: 1.2 g

Saturated Fat: 0.2 g

Cholesterol: 0 mg

Sodium: 23 mg

Fiber: 10.1 g

Sugar: 33 g

Vitamin A: 14,735 mg

Vitamin C: 66 mg

Calcium: 68 mg

Iron: 2 mg

Potassium: 342 mg

Blueberry with a Twist Smoothie

BLUEBERRIES and lime are a wonderful flavor combination even though you don't see them often used together. The banana and stevia will give this a balance of sweet with the tart flavor of lime.

INGREDIENTS

1 large ripe banana

1 cup frozen blueberries

1 teaspoon stevia

1 teaspoon lime juice

1 cup water

4 ice cubes

NUTRITIONAL INFORMATION

Calories: 202

Carbohydrate: 51 g

Protein: 2.2 g

Fat: 1.5 g

Saturated Fat: 0.3 g

Cholesterol: 0 mg

Sodium: 3.1 g

Fiber: 7.7 g

Sugar: 30 g

Vitamin A: 160 IU

Vitamin C: 18.4 mg

Calcium: 19.6 mg

Iron: 0.7 mg

Potassium: 578 mg

Peach Mango Smoothie

STUDIES SUGGEST that cinnamon may interfere with your body's absorption of sugars, which means cinnamon may decrease the number of calories your body absorbs. Honey is always a better choice than sugar as a sweetener, and advocates of honey suggest that its amino acid content can increase metabolism.

INGREDIENTS

1 peach
½ cup mango
¼ cup orange juice
1 teaspoon honey
½ teaspoon cinnamon
8 ice cubes

NUTRITIONAL INFORMATION

Calories: 152	Fiber: 3.8 g
Carbohydrate: 39 g	Sugar: 34 g
Protein: 1.8 g	Vitamin A: 4,826 IU
Fat: 0.6 g	Vitamin C: 70 mg
Saturated Fat: 0 g	Calcium: 24 mg
Cholesterol: 0 mg	Iron: 0.3 mg
Sodium: 0.06 mg	Potassium: 486 mg

NannerNilla Smoothie

VANILLA provides aromatherapy to reduce cravings for sweets. The massive amount of delicious and healthy fruits will satisfy any other cravings you may have.

INGREDIENTS
½ cup blueberries
½ cup apple juice
½ teaspoon vanilla extract
½ cup frozen strawberries
½ frozen banana
Water (optional as needed)

NUTRITIONAL INFORMATION

Calories: 197
Carbohydrate: 49 g
Protein: 1.7 g
Fat: 0.6 g
Saturated Fat: 0.1 g
Cholesterol: 0 mg
Sodium: 7.4 mg

Fiber: 5.6 g
Sugar: 33 g
Vitamin A: 128 IU
Vitamin C: 109 mg
Calcium: 34 mg
Iron: 1.7 mg
Potassium: 581 mg

8

Detox Smoothies

IF YOU SKIPPED to this chapter you may have missed guidelines provided at the beginning of the Weight Loss Smoothies chapter on page 69. Take a minute and read our suggestions on making the perfect smoothie.

Don't feel like turning back to read directions? Well, here is a quick summary:

Add your ingredients in this order:

1. Liquids

2. Semisolids

3. Fruit

4. Frozen Fruit

5. Ice

When blending start slow and wait until the ingredients are circulating easily and then increase power for about 45 seconds. If you want a lighter smoothie with more air, let it blend on high for another 45 seconds. Enjoy.

Raw Fruity Tootie

KALE is one of the most nutritious vegetables on earth. Kale is an excellent source of vitamins A, C, and K, as well as calcium, folate, and potassium. Strawberries, banana, and avocado are all full of fiber, which is great for the colon.

INGREDIENTS
1 cup kale (leaves only)
½ cup water or ice
¼ ripe avocado
½ ripe banana
1 cup strawberries

NUTRITIONAL INFORMATION

Calories: 215

Carbohydrate: 36 g

Protein: 4.8 g

Fat: 8.6 g

Saturated Fat: 1.3 g

Cholesterol: 0 mg

Sodium: 34 mg

Fiber: 9.2 g

Sugar: 14.9 g

Vitamin A: 10,431 IU

Vitamin C: 180 mg

Calcium: 124 mg

Iron: 2.2 mg

Potassium: 987 mg

Sneaky Watermelon

LEMON HELPS the liver by stimulating the release of enzymes, and watermelon has a high concentration of water.

INGREDIENTS

2 leaves organic romaine lettuce
1 banana
1 cup watermelon
1 tablespoon lemon juice

NUTRITIONAL INFORMATION

Calories: 170

Carbohydrate: 43 g

Protein: 3.3 g

Fat: 0.6 g

Saturated Fat: 0.1 g

Cholesterol: 0 mg

Sodium: 12.9 mg

Fiber: 5.8 g

Sugar: 25 g

Vitamin A: 7,955 IU

Vitamin C: 48 mg

Calcium: 38 mg

Iron: 1.4 mg

Potassium: 614 mg

Classic Green Detox Smoothie

KALE is loaded with fiber, and an apple a day truly can keep the doctor away. The ginger root keeps your stomach calm while it digests all that fiber, but make sure you drink plenty of water!

INGREDIENTS

4 leaves kale

1 apple

1 banana

1 teaspoon ground ginger

¾ cup water

NUTRITIONAL INFORMATION

Calories: 239

Carbohydrate: 60 g

Protein: 4.2 g

Fat: 1.3 g

Saturated Fat: 0.3 g

Cholesterol: 0 mg

Sodium: 32 mg

Fiber: 9 g

Sugar: 33 g

Vitamin A: 10,478 IU

Vitamin C: 99 mg

Calcium: 109 mg

Iron: 1.8 mg

Potassium: 941 mg

Happy Day Green Smoothie

DANDELIONS help break down fat, and parsley is a natural diuretic that helps the body eliminate toxins gently. Cranberries help to fight bacteria in the kidneys, urinary tract, and bladder, and blueberries are loaded with antioxidants.

INGREDIENTS

¼ cup fresh parsley

¼ cup dandelion greens

¼ cup blueberries

¼ cup cranberries

½ cup water

1 small apple

NUTRITIONAL INFORMATION

Calories: 123

Carbohydrate: 32 g

Protein: 1.7 g

Fat: 0.6 g

Saturated Fat: 0 g

Cholesterol: 0 mg

Sodium: 21 mg

Fiber: 6.8 g

Sugar: 20 g

Vitamin A: 2,782 IU

Vitamin C: 39 mg

Calcium: 60 mg

Iron: 1.7 mg

Potassium: 349 mg

Simple Smoothie Detox

GRAPEFRUIT contains lycopene—a powerful antioxidant that may help prevent cancer. It also helps to reduce bad cholesterol by helping keep arteries clear. Apple helps remove metals from your system and, in addition to being full of fiber, helps purify the kidneys and liver.

INGREDIENTS
½ whole red grapefruit
½ apple
1 banana
1 cup dandelion greens
¼ cup water

NUTRITIONAL INFORMATION

Calories: 229

Carbohydrate: 58 g

Protein: 4 g

Fat: 1.2 g

Saturated Fat: 0.2 g

Cholesterol: 0 mg

Sodium: 44 mg

Fiber: 9.2 g

Sugar: 33 g

Vitamin A: 7,128 IU

Vitamin C: 72 mg

Calcium: 141 mg

Iron: 2.2 mg

Potassium: 904 mg

Glowing Skin Smoothie

ANTIOXIDANTS found in berries can help counter free-radical damage, which also helps your skin fight the aging process. Berries also aid in controlling blood sugar, and the flax and avocado contain omega-3 fatty acids, which are good for the skin and also help fight inflammation.

INGREDIENTS

2 teaspoons ground flaxseed
2 teaspoons wheat germ
½ avocado
7 strawberries
½ cup cherries
½ cup blueberries
4 ice cubes

NUTRITIONAL INFORMATION

Calories: 410

Carbohydrate: 51 g

Protein: 13.1 g

Fat: 21 g

Saturated Fat: 2.9 g

Cholesterol: 0 mg

Sodium: 11.6 mg

Fiber: 17.5 g

Sugar: 22 g

Vitamin A: 263 IU

Vitamin C: 72 mg

Calcium: 68 mg

Iron: 4.3 mg

Potassium: 1,125 mg

Blue and Red Detox Smoothie

RAW RED CABBAGE is a cancer-fighting food full of vitamin A and beta-carotene. The chia seeds are full of good fats, while the blueberries are packed with antioxidants.

INGREDIENTS

6 ounces water

2 teaspoons chia seeds, soaked

2 bananas

1 cup blueberries

2 cups chopped raw red cabbage

NUTRITIONAL INFORMATION

Calories: 418

Carbohydrate: 95 g

Protein: 9.3 g

Fat: 6.1 g

Saturated Fat: 0.3 g

Cholesterol: 0 mg

Sodium: 52 mg

Fiber: 19.3 g

Sugar: 50 g

Vitamin A: 2,216 IU

Vitamin C: 139 mg

Calcium: 201 mg

Iron: 3.8 mg

Potassium: 1,389 mg

Green and Orange Goodness

PARSLEY HELPS flush the kidneys, plus it supports liver functions. Mango helps cleanse the colon, and the orange juice makes it all taste sunny and delicious.

INGREDIENTS

1 cup fresh parsley
1 large mango
1 cup ice
6 ounces orange juice

NUTRITIONAL INFORMATION

Calories: 233	Fiber: 6 g
Carbohydrate: 57 g	Sugar: 45 g
Protein: 4.1 g	Vitamin A: 6,978 IU
Fat: 1.4 g	Vitamin C: 222 mg
Saturated Fat: 0.2 g	Calcium: 122 mg
Cholesterol: 0 mg	Iron: 4.3 mg
Sodium: 39 mg	Potassium: 996 mg

Roma Detox

TOMATOES contain lycopene, which is a cancer fighter, and the dandelion greens are great for breaking down fat and releasing bile from the gallbladder. Bye bye bile.

INGREDIENTS

1 cup dandelion greens
3 Roma tomatoes
1½ cups water

NUTRITIONAL INFORMATION

Calories: 65

Carbohydrate: 14.1 g

Protein: 3.5 g

Fat: 0.9 g

Saturated Fat: 0.1 g

Cholesterol: 0 mg

Sodium: 57 mg

Fiber: 3.9 g

Sugar: 5.4 g

Vitamin A: 6,839 IU

Vitamin C: 55 mg

Calcium: 103 mg

Iron: 2.4 mg

Potassium: 628 mg

Pomberry Smoothie

POMEGRANATE has more antioxidants than green tea and provides a distinct, tangy flavor. High in vitamin C and antioxidant B vitamins, this smoothie will benefit your health by boosting your immune system as well as providing help in detoxing your body.

INGREDIENTS

1 cup mixed frozen berries
½ cup unsweetened pomegranate juice
½ cup water

NUTRITIONAL INFORMATION

Calories: 155

Carbohydrate: 39 g

Protein: 1.3 g

Fat: 0 g

Saturated Fat: 0 g

Cholesterol: 0 mg

Sodium: 10 mg

Fiber: 5.3 g

Sugar: 32 g

Vitamin A: 0 IU

Vitamin C: 41 mg

Calcium: 37 mg

Iron: 2 g

Potassium: 220 mg

Kale Green Smoothie

KALE IS RECOGNIZED for providing support for the body's detoxification system. Research has shown that isothiocyanates made from kale's glucosinolates can help regulate detox at a genetic level. A bunch of big words that mean kale does a body good.

INGREDIENTS

1 cup firmly packed, stems removed kale or collard greens

½ Granny Smith apple

1 ripe banana

¼ cup loosely packed fresh flat-leaf parsley leaves

1 cup water

NUTRITIONAL INFORMATION

Calories: 184

Carbohydrate: 46 g

Protein: 4 g

Fat: 1 g

Saturated Fat: 0.2 g

Cholesterol: 0 mg

Sodium: 38 mg

Fiber: 7.4 g

Sugar: 23 g

Vitamin A: 11,691 IU

Vitamin C: 117 mg

Calcium: 127 mg

Iron: 2.5 mg

Potassium: 805 mg

South Seas Smoothie

JUST LIKE REGULAR WATER, coconut water helps detox your body by flushing out harmful bacteria and keeping you hydrated. Coconut water helps you stay hydrated because it's an excellent source of electrolytes, and one 8.5-ounce serving has fifteen times more potassium than most sports drinks. Potassium is one of the electrolytes that helps your body replace and retain the fluids needed to operate most efficiently.

INGREDIENTS

1 cup mango chunks
1 tablespoon lime juice
1 cup unsweetened coconut water
Pinch of cayenne powder

NUTRITIONAL INFORMATION

Calories: 154

Carbohydrate: 37 g

Protein: 2.5 g

Fat: 1 g

Saturated Fat: 0.5 g

Cholesterol: 0 mg

Sodium: 255 mg

Fiber: 5.6 g

Sugar: 31 g

Vitamin A: 1,565 IU

Vitamin C: 53 mg

Calcium: 75 mg

Iron: 0.9 mg

Potassium: 863 mg

Orange Double-Berry Smoothie

CITRUS FRUITS are very acidic, and acidic fruits are excellent for helping the body detox. Oranges, while being acidic, are also high in vitamin C, and the fiber they provide is necessary for healthy elimination.

INGREDIENTS

1 navel orange
½ cup frozen blueberries
½ cup frozen raspberries
¼ cup water

NUTRITIONAL INFORMATION

Calories: 155

Carbohydrate: 38 g

Protein: 2.3 g

Fat: 0.5 g

Saturated Fat: 0 g

Cholesterol: 0 mg

Sodium: 0.8 mg

Fiber: 11.6 g

Sugar: 24 g

Vitamin A: 236 IU

Vitamin C: 90 mg

Calcium: 86 mg

Iron: 1.2 mg

Potassium: 302 mg

Green Dew
Mint Smoothie

CUCUMBERS work as a detox aid, facilitating excretion of wastes through the kidneys, thus avoiding the body's need to purge waste through the skin. In other words, cucumbers are good for your healthy skin, too.

INGREDIENTS
¼ cucumber, peeled
1 cup honeydew melon
½ cup pear juice
1 tablespoon fresh lime juice
⅛ cup fresh mint leaves

NUTRITIONAL INFORMATION

Calories: 218	Fiber: 1.8 g
Carbohydrate: 52 g	Sugar: 38 g
Protein: 2.1 g	Vitamin A: 127 IU
Fat: 0.4 g	Vitamin C: 87 mg
Saturated Fat: 0.1 g	Calcium: 18.3 mg
Cholesterol: 0 mg	Iron: 1.1 mg
Sodium: 33 mg	Potassium: 478 mg

Tummy Buddy Smoothie

GINGER helps speed up your circulation, promoting healthy sweating and supporting liver function, therefore helping your body in its efforts to detoxify.

INGREDIENTS

¾ cup papaya
¾ cup sliced peaches
½ pear
1 teaspoon peeled, grated ginger root
4 mint leaves
¼ cup water

NUTRITIONAL INFORMATION

Calories: 148
Carbohydrate: 37 g
Protein: 2.5 g
Fat: 0.7 g
Saturated Fat: 0.1 g
Cholesterol: 0 mg
Sodium: 4.6 mg

Fiber: 6.6 g
Sugar: 25 g
Vitamin A: 1,586 IU
Vitamin C: 77 mg
Calcium: 43 mg
Iron: 0.7 mg
Potassium: 635 mg

Flax to the Max Smoothie

FOODS RICH in omega-3 fatty acids like flaxseed and avocado can aid in the detoxification process by lubricating your intestinal walls, absorbing unhealthy toxins, and then helping to remove those toxins from your body.

INGREDIENTS

½ cup blueberries

½ cup pitted cherries

¼ avocado, peeled

1 teaspoon wheat germ

2 teaspoons ground flaxseed

¼ cup water

NUTRITIONAL INFORMATION

Calories: 220

Carbohydrate: 30 g

Protein: 5.1 g

Fat: 10.9 g

Saturated Fat: 1.4 g

Cholesterol: 0 mg

Sodium: 6.1 mg

Fiber: 9.5 g

Sugar: 16.9 g

Vitamin A: 163 IU

Vitamin C: 12.4 mg

Calcium: 38 mg

Iron: 1.7 mg

Potassium: 555 mg

Green Banana Smoothie

SWISS CHARD is a spinach substitute as it has a similar flavor and its leaves blend very well in smoothies. Chard leaves have a salty flavor that works well with the sweet tastes of fruits you add to your smoothie.

INGREDIENTS
2 bananas
Handful of Swiss chard leaves,
    stems removed
Handful of kale leaves
½ cup almond milk

NUTRITIONAL INFORMATION

Calories: 250	Fiber: 7.6 g
Carbohydrate: 59 g	Sugar: 29 g
Protein: 4.5 g	Vitamin A: 6,653 IU
Fat: 2.5 g	Vitamin C: 66 mg
Saturated Fat: 0.3 g	Calcium: 166 mg
Cholesterol: 0 mg	Iron: 1.7 mg
Sodium: 145 mg	Potassium: 1,158 mg

Sweet Pumpkin Smoothie

PUMPKIN SEEDS combat parasites that live in the digestive tract and also help the liver cleanse toxins from your body. Pumpkin seeds contain antioxidants that fight oxidative damage and in doing so protect your liver.

INGREDIENTS

½ cup mango cubes
½ cup cantaloupe cubes
½ cup fresh pineapple cubes
¼ cup chopped pumpkin seeds
¼ cup water

NUTRITIONAL INFORMATION

Calories: 283
Carbohydrate: 35 g
Protein: 10.5 g
Fat: 12.5 g
Saturated Fat: 2.7 g
Cholesterol: 0 mg
Sodium: 27 mg

Fiber: 4.4 g
Sugar: 27 g
Vitamin A: 3,669 IU
Vitamin C: 93 mg
Calcium: 26 mg
Iron: 3.2 mg
Potassium: 450 mg

Beta Beauty Smoothie

BETA-CAROTENE is a natural carotenoid, which the body converts into vitamin A, as it needs it. As an antioxidant, beta-carotene cleans up free radicals, reducing oxidation and repairing damaged cells.

INGREDIENTS

½ cup cantaloupe cubes

½ cup papaya

1 orange

2 carrots

¼ inch fresh ginger, peeled

NUTRITIONAL INFORMATION

Calories: 176

Carbohydrate: 43 g

Protein: 3.5 g

Fat: 0.8 g

Saturated Fat: 0.2 g

Cholesterol: 0 mg

Sodium: 101 mg

Fiber: 8.6 g

Sugar: 29 g

Vitamin A: 24,435 IU

Vitamin C: 153 mg

Calcium: 118 mg

Iron: 0.8 mg

Potassium: 1,044 mg

A+ Antioxidant Smoothie

THIS POWERFUL antioxidant smoothie gets a considerable boost with pomegranate seeds, lending a hand toward detoxing the liver. They also boost the immune system, which aids in the defense of the body from harmful toxins.

INGREDIENTS
⅓ cup blueberries
⅓ cup raspberries
⅓ cup pomegranate seeds
1 banana

NUTRITIONAL INFORMATION

Calories: 204
Carbohydrate: 51 g
Protein: 2.7 g
Fat: 0.9 g
Saturated Fat: 0.1 g
Cholesterol: 0 mg
Sodium: 2.1 mg

Fiber: 7.5 g
Sugar: 27 g
Vitamin A: 115 IU
Vitamin C: 30 mg
Calcium: 19.1 mg
Iron: 0.9 mg
Potassium: 522 mg

Pineapple Mango Green Smoothie

THIS ECLECTIC mix of fruits and kale will give you a flavor combination you don't often experience. Kale is well known for its detox support, and adding a handful or two of kale makes this both a delicious and powerful detox smoothie.

INGREDIENTS

½ cup mango
½ cup sliced pineapple
½ cup pineapple juice
1 banana
Handful of kale leaves

NUTRITIONAL INFORMATION

Calories: 265
Carbohydrate: 57 g
Protein: 3.5 g
Fat: 1 g
Saturated Fat: 0.2 g
Cholesterol: 0 mg
Sodium: 20 mg

Fiber: 6.2 g
Sugar: 45 g
Vitamin A: 5,898 IU
Vitamin C: 164 mg
Calcium: 85 mg
Iron: 1.6 mg
Potassium: 887 mg

Avocado Sunrise

AVOCADO IS HIGH in both insoluble and soluble fiber. This is perfect for cleansing the colon and carrying toxins out of the body. Its high fiber content also makes it a good food to lower HDL cholesterol.

INGREDIENTS

½ avocado
½ cup fresh squeezed orange juice
½ cup frozen strawberries
1 banana
¼ cup ice

NUTRITIONAL INFORMATION

Calories: 360	Fiber: 12.4 g
Carbohydrate: 59 g	Sugar: 31 g
Protein: 4.7 g	Vitamin A: 520 IU
Fat: 15.5 g	Vitamin C: 128 mg
Saturated Fat: 2.2 g	Calcium: 49 mg
Cholesterol: 0 mg	Iron: 2 mg
Sodium: 11.6 mg	Potassium: 1,321 mg

Detox Deluxe Smoothie

WALNUTS AND other seeds are a good source of arginine, which aids the liver in removing ammonia, a toxic waste product that occurs during the metabolism of proteins.

INGREDIENTS

1 cup cherries

1 medium orange

2 tablespoons walnuts

⅓ avocado

1 cup fresh spinach

¼ cup water

1 teaspoon honey (optional)

NUTRITIONAL INFORMATION

Calories: 478

Carbohydrate: 57 g

Protein: 9.7 g

Fat: 29 g

Saturated Fat: 3.1 g

Cholesterol: 0 mg

Sodium: 29 mg

Fiber: 13.1 g

Sugar: 41 g

Vitamin A: 3,310 IU

Vitamin C: 94 mg

Calcium: 138 mg

Iron: 2.5 mg

Potassium: 1,150 mg

Tropical Detox Smoothie

CILANTRO has been used as a general detoxifying remedy for years and has been found to chelate (remove) heavy metals like mercury, aluminum, and lead from the body. In fact, it is believed to cross the blood-brain barrier and actually remove those metals from the brain.

INGREDIENTS

Small handful cilantro, with stems
Handful of fresh baby spinach
⅓ cup chopped pineapple
1 small kiwifruit
½ banana
¾ cup water

NUTRITIONAL INFORMATION

Calories: 151

Carbohydrate: 35 g

Protein: 4.4 g

Fat: 0.8 g

Saturated Fat: 0.1 g

Cholesterol: 0 mg

Sodium: 59 mg

Fiber: 5.7 g

Sugar: 21 g

Vitamin A: 5,818 IU

Vitamin C: 123 mg

Calcium: 120 mg

Iron: 2.1 mg

Potassium: 1,083 mg

Tangy Apple Green Smoothie

A HOST OF POWERFUL foods for detoxing makes this a powerful smoothie, full of citrus flavor, which gives your immune system a kick start and helps the body cleanse itself.

INGREDIENTS

2 tangerines
1 apple
1 mango
1 cup dandelion greens
¼ inch fresh ginger, peeled
¾ cup water

NUTRITIONAL INFORMATION

Calories: 347
Carbohydrate: 88 g
Protein: 4.7 g
Fat: 2 g
Saturated Fat: 0.5 g
Cholesterol: 0 mg
Sodium: 52 mg

Fiber: 13.2 g
Sugar: 65 mg
Vitamin A: 8,232 IU
Vitamin C: 123 mg
Calcium: 193 mg
Iron: 3 mg
Potassium: 1,041 mg

Cran+Berry Bliss Smoothie

CRANBERRIES can aid your body's detoxification by cleansing the lymphatic system. The lymphatic system neutralizes waste and carries toxins from your body. Adding lemon juice stimulates the production of glutathione, which is the most important antioxidant the liver depends on during the stages of detoxification.

INGREDIENTS

1 cup mixed frozen berries
1 cup cranberry juice
2 teaspoons peeled, grated ginger root
3 ounces lemon juice

NUTRITIONAL INFORMATION

Calories: 185

Carbohydrate: 48 g

Protein: 2 g

Fat: 0.2 g

Saturated Fat: 0.1 g

Cholesterol: 0 mg

Sodium: 32 mg

Fiber: 6.2 g

Sugar: 26 g

Vitamin A: 24 IU

Vitamin C: 84 mg

Calcium: 77 mg

Iron: 3 mg

Potassium: 322 mg

Almond Berry Smoothie

THIS IS A VERY interesting smoothie, considering ingredients such as almond butter and vanilla, which bring strong flavors to the party. The baby spinach adds chlorophyll to help improve digestion. Spinach also significantly improves liver functioning and vision and reduces blood pressure.

INGREDIENTS

1 cup frozen mixed berries
½ banana
1 cup fresh spinach or baby spinach leaves
1 tablespoon natural almond butter
1 teaspoon vanilla extract
1 cup water

NUTRITIONAL INFORMATION

Calories: 258
Carbohydrate: 38 g
Protein: 5.8 g
Fat: 9.7 g
Saturated Fat: 1 g
Cholesterol: 0 mg
Sodium: 35 mg

Fiber: 7.9 g
Sugar: 22 g
Vitamin A: 2,788 IU
Vitamin C: 48 mg
Calcium: 103 mg
Iron: 2.9 mg
Potassium: 654 mg

Morning Berry Basic

ADDING SPIRULINA gives any smoothie a health kick, as this nutritional supplement aids in the body's natural detoxing. Spirulina can release toxins from the body's cells into the bloodstream and then purge them. The main detoxifying substance in spirulina is chlorophyll, a powerful blood cleanser, which can make a significant improvement in your overall health and potentially lower blood pressure.

INGREDIENTS

2 cups raspberries

1 apple

1 orange

1 tablespoon spirulina powder

4 ice cubes

NUTRITIONAL INFORMATION

Calories: 304

Carbohydrate: 72 g

Protein: 8.7 g

Fat: 2.6 g

Saturated Fat: 0.4 g

Cholesterol: 0 mg

Sodium: 78 mg

Fiber: 24 g

Sugar: 42 g

Vitamin A: 514 IU

Vitamin C: 143 mg

Calcium: 133 mg

Iron: 4 mg

Potassium: 899 mg

Green Hawaiian Smoothie

PINEAPPLE HELPS your body detox due to the enzyme bromelain. According to the National Institutes of Health, bromelain is considered a type of cysteine proteinase, an enzyme that helps break down proteins, which means you can use it as a meat tenderizer as well as a delicious fruit flavor in your smoothie.

INGREDIENTS

1 banana

1 cup pineapple

¼ cup pineapple juice

2 tablespoons coconut milk

1 tablespoon spirulina powder

NUTRITIONAL INFORMATION

Calories: 312

Carbohydrate: 61 g

Protein: 7 g

Fat: 8.3 g

Saturated Fat: 6.6 g

Cholesterol: 0 mg

Sodium: 85 mg

Fiber: 6.5 g

Sugar: 39 g

Vitamin A: 330 IU

Vitamin C: 104 mg

Calcium: 49 mg

Iron: 3.6 mg

Potassium: 863 mg

Green Banana Strikes Back

KIWIFRUIT ADDS a tangy kick and a beautiful green hue to this smoothie, which is full of vitamin C. Grapes stop the formation of mucous in the stomach and are good cleansers for the liver, intestines, and kidneys.

INGREDIENTS

1 banana
2 kiwifruits
½ cup red seedless grapes
⅓ cup apple juice

NUTRITIONAL INFORMATION

Calories: 319

Carbohydrate: 79 g

Protein: 3.4 g

Fat: 1.5 g

Saturated Fat: 0.1 g

Cholesterol: 0 mg

Sodium: 3.7 mg

Fiber: 7.2 mg

Sugar: 39 g

Vitamin A: 76 IU

Vitamin C: 155 mg

Calcium: 92 mg

Iron: 1.3 mg

Potassium: 1,000 mg

Papaya Pure

PAPAYA CAN be difficult to find out of season; they are in season from June to September but are often overlooked as a smoothie ingredient. Loaded with vitamin C and fiber, they help the body fight toxins and clean the colon.

INGREDIENTS

2 papayas
1 banana
Juice of ½ lime
½ cup apple juice
4 ice cubes

NUTRITIONAL INFORMATION

Calories: 376
Carbohydrate: 95 g
Protein: 5.1 g
Fat: 1.4 g
Saturated Fat: 0.4 g
Cholesterol: 0 mg
Sodium: 22 mg

Fiber: 14.2 g
Sugar: 57 g
Vitamin A: 6,737 IU
Vitamin C: 392 mg
Calcium: 159 mg
Iron: 1.1 mg
Potassium: 2,081 mg

Papaya Melon Smoothie

TROPICAL FRUITS, including the tasty papaya, make up a very flavorful smoothie, rich with vitamins and fiber for a detox pick-me-up.

INGREDIENTS

½ papaya
1 cup pineapple chunks
1 cup watermelon
1 banana
¼ cup pineapple juice
4 ice cubes

NUTRITIONAL INFORMATION

Calories: 391
Carbohydrate: 99 g
Protein: 3.3 g
Fat: 0.8 g
Saturated Fat: 0.2 g
Cholesterol: 0 mg
Sodium: 31 mg

Fiber: 7.6 g
Sugar: 71 g
Vitamin A: 3,140 IU
Vitamin C: 255 mg
Calcium: 63 mg
Iron: 2 mg
Potassium: 1,363 mg

Green Melon Sensation

A FRUIT COMBINATION you don't often see, but you will absolutely love. The lime adds a boost of flavor as well as providing great cleansing benefits. Pears contain the antioxidant and anticarcinogen glutathione, which is recommended for the prevention of high blood pressure.

INGREDIENTS

½ cantaloupe melon

2 kiwifruits

1 pear

Juice of ½ lime

¼ cup apple juice

NUTRITIONAL INFORMATION

Calories: 324

Carbohydrate: 81 g

Protein: 5 g

Fat: 1.8 g

Saturated Fat: 0.1 g

Cholesterol: 0 mg

Sodium: 48 mg

Fiber: 11.9 g

Sugar: 61 g

Vitamin A: 9,383 IU

Vitamin C: 259 mg

Calcium: 127 mg

Iron: 1.8 mg

Potassium: 1,510 mg

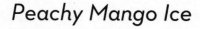

Peachy Mango Ice

THE MANGO and the peach were made for each other and adding them already frozen makes for a very, very cool treat! The Swiss chard leaves make this a very good green smoothie for aiding your detox.

INGREDIENTS

1 frozen mango
1 cup frozen and chopped peaches
¼ cup orange juice
1 handful Swiss chard leaves,
    stems removed

NUTRITIONAL INFORMATION

Calories: 231

Carbohydrate: 59 g

Protein: 3.7 g

Fat: 1.1 g

Saturated Fat: 0 g

Cholesterol: 0 mg

Sodium: 77 mg

Fiber: 7.3 g

Sugar: 51 g

Vitamin A: 10,880 IU

Vitamin C: 113 mg

Calcium: 55 mg

Iron: 1.2 mg

Potassium: 903 mg

Sweet and Sour Smoothie

ACCORDING TO scientific research, milk thistle may protect the cells of the liver by blocking toxins and helping remove them from liver cells. Like other bioflavonoids, milk thistle is a powerful antioxidant, which works to maintain health and energy by protecting the body from damage caused by free radicals that attack healthy cells. In other words, milk thistle can help protect you from cellular deterioration and breakdown seen in aging, like wrinkles, diabetes, coronary artery disease, depression of the immune system, and even cancer.

INGREDIENTS

1 orange
1 nectarine
Juice of 1 lime
2 peaches
4 broccoli florets
4 ice cubes
Milk thistle (see label for
    correct liquid dosage)

(continues)

Sweet and Sour Smoothie (continued)

NUTRITIONAL INFORMATION

Calories: 178

Carbohydrate: 43 g

Protein: 6 g

Fat: 1.3 g

Saturated Fat: 0 g

Cholesterol: 0 mg

Sodium: 30 mg

Fiber: 7.8 g

Sugar: 30 g

Vitamin A: 1,678 IU

Vitamin C: 111 mg

Calcium: 7 mg

Iron: 1.5 mg

Potassium: 980 mg

Apple Sunshine High

FULL OF POWERFUL antioxidants and malic acid, a most potent detoxifier of aluminum, this smoothie is a simple but effective aid in detoxing. Remember, doing a simple detox for even a short period of time is one of the best natural cures for fatigue and excessive tiredness. Help yourself to a smoothie rather than your morning coffee.

INGREDIENTS

1 orange
½ cup nonfat plain yogurt
1 cup unsweetened applesauce
1 teaspoon psyllium seed powder
4 ice cubes

NUTRITIONAL INFORMATION

Calories: 273
Carbohydrate: 65 g
Protein: 4.5 g
Fat: 0.2 g
Saturated Fat: 0 g
Cholesterol: 3.3 mg
Sodium: 282 mg

Fiber: 10.1 g
Sugar: 49 g
Vitamin A: 795 IU
Vitamin C: 75 mg
Calcium: 186 mg
Iron: 3.4 mg
Potassium: 467 mg

Purple Pleasure

PURPLE IS A beautiful color and, in this case, a very healthy color. This recipe is high in vitamin B_{12} and folic acid, which are essential for assisting the body's detoxification. Purple grapes are best for detox as they are particularly good for detoxifying the liver and kidneys. They contain anthocyanins, flavonoids, and resveratrol, which all aid the heart.

INGREDIENTS

1 cup purple grape juice
½ cup blueberries
½ cup orange juice
1 banana
1 tablespoon brewer's yeast

NUTRITIONAL INFORMATION

Calories: 432

Carbohydrate: 98 g

Protein: 9.7 g

Fat: 1.9 g

Saturated Fat: 0.1 g

Cholesterol: 0 mg

Sodium: 28 mg

Fiber: 8.6 g

Sugar: 72 g

Vitamin A: 363 IU

Vitamin C: 139 mg

Calcium: 24 mg

Iron: 5.3 mg

Potassium: 732 mg

Cinnamon Pear Sweetness

IF YOU HAVEN'T TRIED the combination of pears and cinnamon, you are missing out—they are one of nature's great flavor combos, with the "sweet" benefit of being good for you. Pears are high in fiber and "sweep" the body, cleaning the colon to allow the body easier cleansing and elimination. Cinnamon may prevent the accumulation of some fats.

INGREDIENTS

2 pears
½ cup orange juice
1 teaspoon ground cinnamon
1 teaspoon honey

NUTRITIONAL INFORMATION

Calories: 278

Carbohydrate: 73 g

Protein: 2.2 g

Fat: 0.7 g

Saturated Fat: 0 g

Cholesterol: 0 mg

Sodium: 4.5 mg

Fiber: 10.6 g

Sugar: 51 g

Vitamin A: 324 IU

Vitamin C: 76 mg

Calcium: 44 mg

Iron: 0.9 mg

Potassium: 643 mg

Pear Apple Snap

PEARS AND APPLES are a wonderful flavor combination and a great duo for helping the body detox. Psyllium is bulk forming, so it collects water, expands, and "scrubs" down the sides of the intestinal system. Ginger encourages healthy sweating.

INGREDIENTS

2 pears
½ apple
½ cup apple juice
1 teaspoon psyllium seed powder
1 ounce fresh ginger, peeled and crushed

NUTRITIONAL INFORMATION

Calories: 337
Carbohydrate: 86 g
Protein: 2.5 g
Fat: 0 g
Saturated Fat: 0 g
Cholesterol: 0 g
Sodium: 10.6 mg

Fiber: 13.5 g
Sugar: 60 g
Vitamin A: 50 IU
Vitamin C: 68 mg
Calcium: 56 mg
Iron: 1.1 mg
Potassium: 728 mg

Green Tea Goodness

GREEN TEA contains bioflavonoids. Flavonoids are antioxidants, responsible for the many health benefits of green tea. They are potent free-radical scavengers, which help detoxify the body and eliminate the damage done by the free radicals. Besides being a wonderful detox aid, a touch of molasses adds sweetness to this smoothie!

INGREDIENTS

1 cup frozen white grapes

1 cup fresh baby spinach

6 ounces strong brewed green tea, cooled

½ medium avocado

1 teaspoon molasses

NUTRITIONAL INFORMATION

Calories: 258

Carbohydrate: 32 g

Protein: 4.1 g

Fat: 15 g

Saturated Fat: 2.2 g

Cholesterol: 0 mg

Sodium: 47 mg

Fiber: 8 g

Sugar: 22 g

Vitamin A: 2,989 IU

Vitamin C: 16.8 mg

Calcium: 141 mg

Iron: 3.3 mg

Potassium: 1,227 mg

Fruity Dandelion Smoothie

DANDELION stimulates the gall bladder, encouraging the body to break down fat. It's a diuretic; so make sure you drink plenty of water!

INGREDIENTS

½ ripe peach
½ fresh mango
¼ cup apple
1 cup fresh dandelion greens
¼ cup water

NUTRITIONAL INFORMATION

Calories: 126
Carbohydrate: 32 g
Protein: 2.6 g
Fat: 0.8 g
Saturated Fat: 0.1 g
Cholesterol: 0 g
Sodium: 42 mg

Fiber: 5.7 g
Sugar: 24 g
Vitamin A: 9,656 IU
Vitamin C: 54 mg
Calcium: 115 mg
Iron: 1.7 mg
Potassium: 507 mg

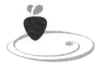

Metric Conversions

The recipes in this book have not been tested with metric measurements, so some variations might occur.

Remember that the weight of dry ingredients varies according to the volume or density factor: 1 cup of flour weighs far less than 1 cup of sugar, and 1 tablespoon doesn't necessarily hold 3 teaspoons.

GENERAL FORMULA FOR METRIC CONVERSION

Ounces to grams	multiply ounces by 28.35
Grams to ounces	multiply ounces by 0.035
Pounds to grams	multiply pounds by 453.5
Pounds to kilograms	multiply pounds by 0.45
Cups to liters	multiply cups by 0.24
Fahrenheit to Celsius	subtract 32 from Fahrenheit temperature, multiply by 5, divide by 9
Celsius to Fahrenheit	multiply Celsius temperature by 9, divide by 5, add 32

VOLUME (LIQUID)
MEASUREMENTS

1 teaspoon = ⅙ fluid ounce = 5 milliliters

1 tablespoon = ½ fluid ounce = 15 milliliters

2 tablespoons = 1 fluid ounce = 30 milliliters

¼ cup = 2 fluid ounces = 60 milliliters

⅓ cup = 2⅔ fluid ounces = 79 milliliters

½ cup = 4 fluid ounces = 118 milliliters

1 cup or ½ pint = 8 fluid ounces = 250 milliliters

2 cups or 1 pint = 16 fluid ounces = 500 milliliters

4 cups or 1 quart = 32 fluid ounces = 1,000 milliliters

1 gallon = 4 liters

VOLUME (DRY)
MEASUREMENTS

¼ teaspoon = 1 milliliter

½ teaspoon = 2 milliliters

¾ teaspoon = 4 milliliters

1 teaspoon = 5 milliliters

1 tablespoon = 15 milliliters

¼ cup = 59 milliliters

⅓ cup = 79 milliliters

½ cup = 118 milliliters

⅔ cup = 158 milliliters

¾ cup = 177 milliliters

1 cup = 225 milliliters

4 cups or 1 quart = 1 liter

½ gallon = 2 liters

1 gallon = 4 liters

WEIGHT (MASS) MEASUREMENTS

1 ounce = 30 grams

2 ounces = 55 grams

3 ounces = 85 grams

4 ounces = ¼ pound = 125 grams

8 ounces = ½ pound = 240 grams

12 ounces = ¾ pound = 375 grams

16 ounces = 1 pound = 454 grams

LINEAR MEASUREMENTS

½ in = 1½ cm

1 inch = 2½ cm

6 inches = 15 cm

8 inches = 20 cm

10 inches = 25 cm

12 inches = 30 cm

20 inches = 50 cm

OVEN TEMPERATURE EQUIVALENTS, FAHRENHEIT (F) AND CELSIUS (C)

100°F = 38°C

200°F = 95°C

250°F = 120°C

300°F = 150°C

350°F = 180°C

400°F = 205°C

450°F = 230°C

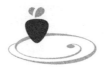

Index